Bone Metastases

Springer
London
Berlin
Heidelberg
New York
Barcelona
Hong Kong
Milan
Paris
Singapore
Tokyo

Dominique G. Poitout (Ed.)

Bone Metastases

Medical, Surgical and Radiological Treatment

With 36 Figures

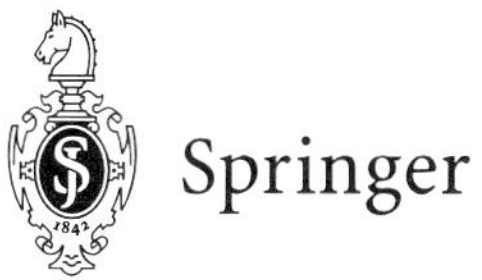

Springer

Dominique G. Poitout, MD, Prof. Chief of Dept.
Service de Chirurgie Orthopédique et de Traumatologie,
Centre Hospitalier Nord, Chemin des Bourrely, 13915 Marseille Cedex 20,
France

British Library Cataloguing in Publication Data
Bone metastases: medical, surgical and radiological treatment
1. Bone metastasis - Treatment 2. Bone metastasis - Surgery
I. Poitout, Dominique G.
616.9′9471′06
ISBN 1852334959

Library of Congress Cataloging-in-Publication Data
Bone metastases: medical, surgical and radiological treatment / Dominique Poitout (ed.).
p.; cm.
Includes bibliographical references and index.
ISBN 1-85233-495-9 (alk. paper)
1. Bones–Cancer–Surgery. 2. Bones–Cancer–Treatment. 3. Metastasis–Treatment.
I. Poitout, Dominique G.
[DNLM: 1. Bone Neoplasms–secondary. 2. Bone Neoplasms–drug therapy. 3. Bone Neoplasms–radiotherapy. 4. Orthopedic Procedures. WE 258 B7108 2002]
RD675.B657 2002
616.99′47106–dc21 2001040002

ISBN 1-85233-495-9 Springer-Verlag London Berlin Heidelberg
a member of BertelsmannSpringer Science+Business Media GmbH
http: //www. springer. co.uk

Printed in Great Britain

Typeset by Expo Holdings Sdn Bhd, Kuala Lumpur, Malaysia
Printed and bound at the Cromwell Press, Trowbridge, Wiltshire
28/3830-543210 Printed on acid-free paper SPIN 10835635

Foreword

by Professor Antonie H.M. Taminiau

As the population becomes older, it might be expected that the incidence of cancer will increase and that cancer will be the main cause of death in the near future. Based on the incidence patterns, the risk (life table method) of developing cancer before the age of 75 years is about 25% for males and females. If the incidence pattern is maintained, nearly four out of ten men and 3.5 out of ten women will get cancer during their lives. The majority of these patients will be over 45 years of age. Less than 10% of all new cancer patients are younger than 45 years and children seldom develop cancer. Treatment of primary cancer, depending on the type and stage of the disease, may cure the patient. When the cancer has metastasised, however, the possibility of cure is generally limited and therefore attention should be focussed more on quality of life than on survival. Bone metastases may seriously affect this quality of life.

The incidence of bone metastases in cancer patients is reported to be as high as 30–70%. More than 80% of these are due to carcinoma of the breast, prostate, lung or kidney. The majority of these metastases are predominantly found in the axial skeleton. Bone metastases are often asymptomatic unless soft tissues are involved or fracture occurs. Stabilisation of impending and pathological fractures is the treatment of choice and effects pain relief, restoration of limb function and early mobilisation, and therefore improves the quality of life.

In skeletal metastases the risk of a pathological fracture is related primarily to the degree of tumour extension and of bone destruction. The overall incidence of fractures due to bone metastases is 5–10%.

The development of an impending fracture, pathological fracture or spinal metastases is not necessarily a terminal event. Since the life span of these patients has been extended, proper treatment of the lesions significantly adds to the life quality of the individual patient. Postoperative radiotherapy is an essential part of treatment, as are chemotherapy and hormonal therapy in sensitive car-cinomas.

In this book the multidisciplinary approach for treatment of bone metastases is discussed extensively by all disciplines. The new strategies in medical treatment (chemotherapy, immunotherapy, biphosphonates, hormonal and cement-containing drugs) are illuminated. The role and interaction of radiotherapy and surgery of long bones and spine are discussed. Spinal decompression and stabilisation are increasingly important in metastatic disease. This book is an excellent state-of-the-art summary of all the aspects concerning bone metastases and will serve as a guideline for any doctor confronted with the problems of these patients.

Antonie H.M. Taminiau,
Orthopaedic Oncology,
Leiden University Medical Centre,
The Netherlands

Foreword

by Professor Michel Forest

A metastasis of cancer to bone is a frequent clinical problem, and is often associated with significant morbidity due to osteolysis.

Metastatic bone lesions are much more common than are primary malignant bone tumors, and compromise the patient's health by causing intense pain, osteolysis, pathological fractures, hypercalcemia, and bone marrow replacement,

Much progress has been made recently on the biology of boneresorbing cells and on the understanding of the multistep process of bone metastases that involves interactions between tumor cells and the unique microenvironment of bone.

The management challenge for patients with metastatic bone disease needs, in most cases, a multimodality approach to optimize care and quality of life. This books is the reflect of various treatment modalities, the well established ones as well as new approaches in the fields of orthopedic surgery, radiation therapy, chemotherapy, systemic therapy (endocrine treatment changes and assessment of the use of biphosphonates).

This work includes also important contributions on diagnosis (imaging and pathology), and on the management of palliative care.

This integrated approach is written by authoritative experts in the various fields of diagnosis and treatment, and without any doubt, this relevant and organized text reflecting a great experience on the new improvements and developments of the therapeutic approaches, should be of utmost value for the quality of life of patients requiring often palliative and supporting treatments for many months or sometimes years

Michel Forest, M.D., Professor of Pathology
Hôpital Cochin,
Paris,
France

Preface

This book will discuss the actual approach of Bone Metastases in the fields of diagnosis, medical and surgical treatment.

Bone metastases are frequently one of the first signs of disseminated disease in cancer patients and a major source of morbidity. Skeletal metastases may appear radiographically as osteolytic, osteoblastic or mixed lesions. As a general rule, the radiographic appearance of a skeletal metastasis does not necessarily indicate the primary lesion. However, in some clinical instances, the radiographic findings may be very evocative.

Bone metastases are very frequent but probably underestimated, as shown by studies on iliac crest biopsies. They may be indicative of a clinically silent tumour. The diagnosis is based on biopsies of bone marrow, needle puncture of suspicious zones or surgical biopsies. The spine, skull and pelvis are the most common sites, but the ribs and the epiphysis and metaphysis of long bones may also be affected. Metastases in the distal bones are rare, but are more likely to affect the metatarsal and metacarpal bones than the phalanges. Some tumours (breast, prostate, thyroid, kidney and lung) have specific affinities for the bone tissue. Bone lesions may also occasionally result from endometrial carcinoma. These tumour types arise in endocrine-dependent organs. Tumour development and progression can also be influenced by the hormonal environment.

Bone metastases may occur only in the marrow, they may lead to an osteoblastic appearance. Histologically, the diagnosis is easy if the primary tumour is known, but difficult when the original cancer is silent. In some cases, the pathologist will be able to specify the starting point with certainty. More often, it will only be possible to suggest a diagnosis without confirmation of the origin, unless the metastasis is very differentiated and reproduces the primary tumour (hypernephroma, oat-cell carcinoma of lung, adenocarcinoma of thyroid). In these circumstances, immuno-histochemistry helps to specify the diagnosis. The mechanisms of metastatic growth involve cellular chemotactic factors and connections with the caval venous system at the vertebral level, in the vascular bone network. It is what the optimum systemic treatment for bone metastases depends on the tumour type. Chemotherapy is demonstrably effective in the treatment of bone metastases.

The role of immunotherapy in the treatment of cancer is very limited and restricted to the use of interferon and IL-2. Objective responses in bone metastases have been observed in renal cell cancer and metastatic melanoma.

Biphosphonates represent a major therapeutic advance in the management of tumour-induced osteolysis and skeletal morbidity, successfully treat hypercalcaemic episodes, relieve bone pain and may lead to recalcification of lytic metastases. Prolonged use of clodronate or pamidronate decreases the frequency of skeletal-related events in patients with metastatic bone disease. Another putative role for biphosphonate treatment is the prevention or delaying of the development of bone metastases in breast cancer patients.

Hormonal therapy is aimed at depriving tumours of hormonal stimuli by lowering either oestrogen or androgen levels or by competitively blocking their receptors. New agents that are currently available (anti-oestrogens, anti-aromatases, lutinising hormone-releasing hormone (LH-RH) agonists) have an enlarged spectrum of activity, but also less toxicity. Reduction in tumour volume or inhibition of tumour growth can be consistently obtained and disease-related symptoms relieved in a significant number of treated patients.

External local radiotherapy remains the major treatment of bone metastasis. Radiation therapy is usually performed to relieve local bone pain, to prevent pathological fracture, vertebral collapse, and to promote healing in pathological fracture and relief of spinal cord compression.

External radiotherapy with high-energy photons can be delivered for all bone metastases, as there is no difference of response according to histological type. Results seem to depend on the location of the bone metastases.

Systemic radiation therapy using beta-emitting radionucleotides is used in patients with generalised pain, and give less bone marrow toxicity than hemibody external irradiation. Radiosurgical treatment reduces pain and maintains mobility in patients with an average life expectancy of 10 months. As well as increasing the patient's comfort, radiosurgical treatment allows basic treatment of the illness to be continued.

Surgery for bone metastasis is palliative, with the following aims :

- Suppression of the pain associated with the metastasis
- Prevention of pathological fractures
- Stabilisation of the bone using osteosynthesis or a prosthesis
- Conservation of function, allowing rapid rehabilitation
- Continuation of medical treatment and an early return home.

Vertebral stabilisation and adjuvant treatment have allowed considerable therapeutic progress over recent decades. The best results are obtained when operations are performed before the patient becomes malnourished and before multiple metastatic sites develop. From the surgical point of view, extended excision as total vertebrectomy gives better results than limited surgery.

For long-term survival, control of the tumour is essential. Advances in implant design and surgical techniques have allowed a more aggressive approach to these tumours, with rewarding results.

We have only recently become aware that the sick can think, have emotions and feelings, and that we should accompany them on the psycho-effective path.

All these subjects are developed in the next chapters by specialists of these different topics.

D.G. Poitout

Contents

Part 5 **Surgical Treatment**

Part 6 **Medico-social Aspects**

Part 7 **Pain Relief**

List of Contributors

Dr Richard Aswad
Orthopaedic Surgeon
Upper Extremity Surgery and Microsurgery
Centre Borely Mermoz
114 rue Jean Mermoz
13008 Marseille
France

Dr Marjorie Baciuchka-Palmaro
Department of Oncology
Centre Hospitalier Régional et Universitaire de Marseille
Hôpital de la Timone
264 rue St Pierre
13385 Marseille cedex 05
France

Dr Mireille Chriostine Berthoud
Consultant Anaesthetist
Department of Anaesthesia
Royal Hallamshire Hospital
Glossop Road
Sheffield S10 2JF
UK

Professor Christophe Chagnaud
Department of Radiology
Hôpital de la Conception
147 boulevard Baille
13385 Marseille cedex 05
France

Dr Daniel Chevassut
Psychologist (Ethics)
Department of Orthopaedic Surgery and Trauma
Hôpital Nord
Chemin des Bourrellys
13915 Marseille cedex 20
France

Dr B. Clouet d'Orval
Department of Orthopaedic Surgery and Trauma
Hôpital Nord
Chemin des Bourrellys
13915 Marseille cedex 20
France

Dr Elodie Cretel
Department of Radiotherapy and Oncology
Centre Hospitalier Régional et Universitaire de Marseille
Hôpital de la Timone
264 rue St Pierre
13385 Marseille cedex 05
France

Dr Thierry Dorval
Institut Curie
26 rue d'Ulm
75005 Paris
France

Dr Florence Duffaud
Department of Oncology
Centre Hospitalier Régional et Universitaire de Marseille
Hôpital de la Timone
264 rue St Pierre
13385 Marseille cedex 05
France

Professor Roger Favre
Department of Oncology
Centre Hospitalier Régional et Universitaire de Marseille
Hôpital de la Timone
264 rue St Pierre
13385 Marseille cedex 05
France

Dr Pierre Fumoleau
Centre René Gauducheau,
44805 Saint Herblain
France

Professor Charles S.B. Galasko
Consultant Orthopaedic Surgeon
Department of Orthopaedic Surgery
University of Manchester
Clinical Sciences Building
Hope Hospital
Eccles Old Road
Salford M6 8HD
UK

Dr Louise Garbe-Galanti
Department of Anatomy and Pathology
Hôpital Sainte-Marguerite
270 boulevard de Sainte-Marguerite
13009 Marseille
France

Dr Y. Glard
Department of Orthopaedic Surgery and Trauma
Hôpital Nord
Chemin des Bourrellys
13915 Marseille cedex 20
France

Professor Philippe Hernigou
Orthopaedics Department
Hôpital Henri Mondor
51 avenue du Maréchal de Lattre de Tassigny
94010 Creteil
France

Professor Pierre Juin
Department of Radiotherapy and Oncology
Centre Hospitalier Régional et Universitaire de Marseille
Hôpital de la Timone
264 rue St Pierre
13385 Marseille cedex 05
France

Dr Christian Louis
Orthopaedic Surgeon
Centre Phocea
14 boulevard Gustave Ganay
13009 Marseille
France

Professor René Louis
Department of Orthopaedics and Vertebral Surgery
Hôpital de la Conception
147 boulevard Baille
13385 Marseille cedex 05
France

Dr Jean Louis Mouysset
Department of Oncology
12 rue d'Italie
13100 Aix en Provence
France

Professor Michel Panuel
Department of Radiology
Hôpital Nord
Chemin des Bourrellys
13915 Marseille cedex 20
France

Dr Philippe Petit
Department of Paediatric Radiology
Hôpital Timone-Enfants
13395 Marseille cedex 05
France

Dr Thierry Pignon
Department of Radiotherapy and Oncology
Centre Hospitalier Régional et Universitaire de Marseille
Hôpital de la Timone
264 rue St Pierre
13385 Marseille cedex 05
France

Professor Dominique G. Poitout
Department of Orthopaedic Surgery and Trauma
Hôpital Nord
Chemin des Bourrellys
13915 Marseille cedex 20
France

Dr François Portier
Department of Radiology
Hôpital Nord
Chemin des Bourrellys,
13915 Marseille cedex 20
France

Dr Benoit Ripoll
Department of Orthopaedic Surgery and Trauma
Hôpital Nord
Chemin des Bourrellys
13915 Marseille cedex 20
France

Dr Pierre Soulié
Department of Oncology
Centre René Huguenin
35 rue Dailly
92210 Saint-Cloud
France

Dr David Spiegel
Department of Psychiatry and Behavioral Sciences
Stanford University School of Medicine
Stanford
CA 94305-5544
USA

Mr Jonathon B. Spilsbury
Consultant Spinal Surgeon
Department of Orthopaedic Surgery
University of Manchester
Clinical Sciences Building
Hope Hospital
Eccles Old Road
Salford M6 8HD
UK

Dr Patrick Tropiano
Orthopaedic Surgeon
Department of Orthopaedic Surgery and Trauma
Hôpital Nord
Chemin des Bourrellys
13915 Marseille cedex 20
France

Dr M. Tubiana-Hulin
Department of Oncology
Centre René Huguenin
35 rue Dailly
92210 Saint-Cloud
France

Introduction: Basic Principles of Surgery in Musculoskeletal Oncology

D.G. Poitout and Y. Glard

In everyday practice, the clinical classification of cancers that determines most therapeutic procedures poorly assesses prognosis. However, the unpredictable evolution of the treated tumour may result from discrepancies between clinical classification and biological reality. These discrepancies may account for unexpected and unpredictable therapeutic failures with apparently localised small tumours, as well as for long-term good results with locally advanced tumours.

Chemotherapy

Improvements in the treatment of bone tumours over the past 20 years have led to a significant increase in absolute cure rates. The following drugs have a proven effect on bone tumours of all histological types:

- Alkylating drugs: cyclophosphamid, cisplatin, dacarbazin, mitomycin
- Antimetabolites: methotrexate
- Intercalants: anthracyclin, especially adriamycin, and actinomycin D
- Alkaloids: vincristin (vindesine has a weak effect).

Intra-arterial infusion of cytotoxic agents after arteriography is justified if the tumour is highly vascularised. This procedure increases the plasma drug concentration around the tumour during the infusion. The antitumour effect can be impressive with 24- to 72-hour infusions.

When several afferent pedicles can be isolated, preoperative embolisation of accessory pedicles may complement cytotoxic drug infusion through the main pedicle. Sterilisation rates from this method range from 30 to 40%, but the histological response is greater.

Nowadays, interferon is used to treat viral diseases, as well as malignancy. Outstanding results have been obtained in patients with laryngeal papilloma. Obstructive masses of soft tissue virtually disappear after a short treatment. The treatment must be repeated to obtain a definitive remission.

Radiotherapy

Improvements in Radiotherapy

Improvements in radiotherapy depend on various factors:

- High-power photons: either cobalt photons or 5, 10 or 15 MeV photons from an accelerator allow satisfactory cutaneous protection, better efficiency in deep tissues and a better absorption homogeneity between the bone and the soft tissue
- Electrons are particularly useful in some superficial sites (ribs, sternum, skull) because they spare deep tissues (depending on the selected penetration)
- The biological efficiency of neutrons and heavy ions is higher than that of photons; they are mainly used in radioresistant tumours
- New medical imaging processes have improved the irradiation target volume (computed tomography scanning, nuclear magnetic resonance imaging and isotope imaging).

Radiotherapy Efficiency

The efficiency of radiotherapy has been improved by:

- A new splitting process adjusted to the cellular kinetics of individual tumours: low splitting or high splitting
- New radiochemotherapy combinations: administration of radio- and chemotherapy simultaneously potentiates their individual effects
- Use of radiosensitising drugs, such as flagyl, metronidazol, bromodecoxyuridin
- Physical radiosensitising (thermic rise) localised deep radioactive hyperthermia or regional hyperthermia of a limb with an extracorporeal circulation.

Per-operative Radiotherapy

Per-operative radiotherapy has been recommended for several years to treat tumours that are impossible to remove, such as those of the uterus and pancreas. It is also used as a complement to insufficient resection of some bone tumours of the pelvis (chondrosarcoma or fibrosarcoma).

Half-body Irradiation

Half-body irradiation is commonly used for patients with multiple bone metastases and is sometimes offered as an alternative to chemotherapy for the treatment of radiosensitive tumours, such as lymphoma, myeloma or Ewing's sarcoma.

Full-body Irradiation with Marrow Graft

Commonly used to treat malignant haemopathy, full-body irradiation with marrow graft is offered in some cases of Ewing's sarcoma, particularly multimetastatic and chemoresistant cases.

The use of radiotherapy depends on the histology of the tumour, which determines its radiosensitivity, and whether it is a primary tumour or a bone metastasis.

Surgical Treatment

Biopsy

A biopsy is necessary whenever the diagnosis is uncertain, or if the lesion is malignant, even if the diagnosis has been confirmed. Biopsy is a major surgical procedure that has to be performed perfectly because the credibility of the diagnosis depends on the quality of the performance, and complications are likely to compromise therapeutic opportunities and thus the prognosis. Biopsy must be performed by an experienced surgeon.

Apart from the risks associated with the procedure, spreading of malignant cells is a potential problem. Cartilaginous tumours are able to survive in the operating scars, which must therefore be removed completely. The risk is more hypothetical if we consider general spreading. Circulating malignant cells exist spontaneously and their rate increases more after palpation than after biopsy. The metastatic risk is not linked to the number of cells, but to the host-tumour relationship.

Surgical Biopsy

All clinical, radiological, biological and surgical information must be given to the pathologist for an accurate diagnosis to be made. Although difficult to perform, surgical biopsy is a useful procedure because it allows a macroscopic assessment of the lesion and a controlled selection of the sampling zone.

Procedures for prevention of infection are as follows:

- Aseptic operative theatre
- Strict precautions in the preparation of the operating zone and during the operation
- Antibiotic therapy
- Temporary haemostasis
- Pneumatic tourniquet when possible
- Banning of Esmarch's bandage (at least around the tumour)
- Loosen tourniquet after sampling to check haemostasis.

Blood transfusion is not routine, but should be scheduled in case of haemorrhagic lesions. Instruments include an electric knife and the usual instruments for soft tissue and bones.

A radiograph set on a light box may be used to locate the tumour. Previous radiological location on the skin or use of an intensifier screen may be required.

For lesions in multiple locations, select the one that is easiest to approach. A good view is necessary. Respect the anatomical compartments that will be required to cover the bone at the end of the operation. Avoid regions where the tumour has invaded hypodermic tissues. It should be possible to remove the biopsy scars in a subsequent operation.

Take multiple samples: peripheral to the lesion, include the cortex if it exists, and from several areas within the tumour.

Remove the pneumatic tourniquet when the sampling is finished, to complete haemostasis with the electric knife. Haemorrhage may be perfectly controlled. If there is weeping, close after placing a vacuum drain in the surgical approach. Do not drain if the haemorrhage is substantial. After a long-lasting temporary tamponage, close hermetically to obtain a compressive cover and use a compression dressing.

Postoperatively, the patient will need to be immobilised if the bone is fragile. Postpone the removal of stitches if radiotherapy is being considered.

Complications of surgical biopsy include:

- Taking a biopsy outside the tumour
- Superficial sampling (inexperienced surgeon)
- Indecipherable sampling from a necrotic zone (multiple sampling is necessary)
- Pathological fracture during or after the biopsy (upper extremity or diaphysis of the femur)
- Haematoma
- Infection.

Pathological fracture may be avoided by smooth manipulation during trephining and by preventive postoperative immobilisation. Treatment is by postoperative immobilisation. Haematoma compromises healing of the wound, delays irradiation if needed and may lead to infection. The blood contains tumour cells, which may increase the volume of soft tissue that needs to be removed. Infection may have tragic consequences, leading to amputation in cases where conservative surgery and irradiation may have been possible.

Biopsy with a Trocar

A trocar less than 4 mm diameter is required (if it is greater than 4 mm, there is a risk of uncontrollable haemorrhage or fragile bone fracture), with or without indentation, hand-driven or driven by a variable-speed electric motor.

Accurate location is essential, and an intensifier screen may be needed. Under local anaesthesia, puncture the skin with a bistoury, and drive the trocar down to the bone

If the tumour is poorly ossified, a fast-rotating trocar may be used. If the tumour is very hard, use an indented trocar, hand or mechanically driven, with a slow rotation. Special precautions are needed for biopsy of the vertebrae.

Various procedures can be used for biopsy of the tumour. The direct approach is simple and logical for the posterior wall, but unsuitable for a thoracic or lumbar vertebral body. In the latter, percutaneous puncture biopsies using an intensifier screen should be considered, or, if these fail, transpedicular biopsy. Puncture biopsy is not performed on the cervical vertebrae for safety reasons. It could only be done with a small trocar, which would produce undersized samples. In any case, an anterolateral approach of the cervical vertebrae is easy.

A 3-7 mm diameter trocar is used for percutaneous puncture biopsy of the thoracic and lumbar vertebrae. It is inserted under general anaesthesia and using intensifier screen control, the needle making a 45° angle from a penetration point located on the external edge of the paravertebral muscles, 7-8 cm from the middle of the posterior wall. The trocar then goes between the two transverse apophyses.

Transpedicular biopsy is indicated if the localisation in the vertebral body is difficult to reach by a percutaneous puncture or if the percutaneous puncture fails (for example, a central localisation). It is feasible from C7 to S1. Pedicles are catheterised with a 3 mm drill, then a 4 mm drill, to a depth of 25 mm, to reach the spongy bone of the vertebral body. A straight curette is then passed through to allow sampling.

Advantages and Disadvantages of Trocar Biopsies

A biopsy with a trocar avoids:

- A complex surgical approach (vertebrae)
- Any complication linked to surgery (infection, haemorrhage)
- General anaesthesia
- In some cases, hospitalisation.

However, a biopsy with a trocar does not give as much information as a surgical biopsy. It does not allow any macroscopic selection from the sample, which is a great drawback for polymorphic lesions. If no significant result is obtained from a trocar biopsy, it can be repeated, or a surgical biopsy can be performed. Like any blind procedure, it can lead to specific complications and must be performed with caution in order to avoid inopportune injuries.

Use of Biopsy Samples

Samples are used for classical anatomical and pathological examination. The type of fixation fluid (formol or Bouin) is not important, but it must be of sufficient quantity. Problems include losing the samples, not filling in the examination form and misidentification of the patient.

A pathologist is required in the operating theatre if prints are to be prepared for cytological studies, if samples are to be prepared for electron microscopic studies, and for microbiological examination of samples.

Extemporaneous examination is ineffective in the case of bone pathology because a hard sample may require decalcification. Treatment can be started only in cases where a diagnosis has been confirmed radioclinically. In some rare cases, extemporaneous examination can be useful to control the excision borders of a malignant lesion.

A biopsy can be performed as an isolated procedure, before confirmation of the diagnosis. This should be the rule for primary malignant tumours. The patient should be prepared psychologically while waiting for the diagnosis, particularly if there is a high suspicion of malignancy, which will require further treatment.

A biopsy may also be used in association with therapeutic procedures, during the same operation. Examples include:

- Biopsy excision and biopsy-scrapping out grafts (benign tumours)
- Biopsy and osteosynthesis (fragile benign tumours and bone metastases)
- Biopsy followed by resection and use of prostheses (bone metastases).

Curettage, Resection and Amputation

Curettage

In a curettage, we deliberately get into the tumour, which is scraped out from inside. In an amputation, the limb is sacrificed. In a resection, the limb is spared, but the whole tumour is removed without any penetration of the tumour. The bone segment containing the tumour is removed in a single block with all the soft tissue.

Resection

Resection may be marginal, wide or radical, according to the distance between the incision and the tumour.

In a marginal resection, the tumour can be seen. It is excised around the outside of the capsule or pseudocapsule, without penetrating it. Marginal resection is possible for aggressive benign tumours (some tumours with giant cells), but is unsuitable for malignant tumours.

In a wide resection, a layer of apparently healthy tissue is left around the tumour. Neither the tumour nor its pseudocapsule can be seen. This is an intracompartmental resection. Wide resection is the ideal routine surgery for malignant tumours. The amount of bone and soft tissue removed varies according to the degree of malignancy and the clarity of the tumour limits.

In a radical resection, anatomical compartments that are not affected by the lesion are removed. This extracompartmental resection is advised only if the tumour has high-grade malignancy, confirmed histologically, and is locally extended, invading the bone segment and its adjacent soft tissue. In our opinion, this type of resection should be exceptional. Wide resections are usually sufficient, even if there is a bad histological prognosis. Experience shows that local relapses are not more frequent with this option.

Contaminated resections and splitting up resections are either operative "mistakes" or deliberate palliative procedures. The surgeon may start a resection, and local difficulties lead him either to penetrate the tumour (contaminated resection) or to split it up to remove it. The procedure is then said to be "non-carcinological". The chances of relapse increase substantially (although they are not as high as those after a curettage). A contaminated resection may be performed as a palliative procedure in special cases where no other treatment is possible, such as excision of a vertebral tumour from the vertebral body and posterior wall, or resection of a huge tumour.

Amputation

Like a resection, an amputation can be radical, wide, marginal or contaminated. Amputation itself does not provide more carcinological security. It is performed only when resection is impossible because of tumour extension, or if resection is likely to sacrifice blood vessels and nerves, or leave a poorly functional limb (paralysed, with ischaemia, shortened, dangling). Amputation may be performed if there has been previous multiple surgery, infection or radiotherapy.

Consequently, it is often the state of the soft tissue and not the state of the bone that leads to amputation.

Bone Grafts

Fresh autografts are the only osteogenic bone grafts. However, taking a massive graft or a large amount of spongy or cortical bone is harmful to the patient. Other risks include a lengthy operation, haematoma, infection, osteitis and cosmetic after-effects. Allografts are therefore used more frequently.

Types of Allograft

Cryopreserved Allografts

Cryopreservation is the most common method. The preservation temperature is not sterilising, so all sources of contamination must be eliminated. Donors must be selected carefully. A previous microbiological investigation is necessary (for bacteria, viruses and fungi). The graft must be taken and handled under aseptic conditions, thus avoiding any secondary contamination.

Biomechanical characteristics of grafts are not altered by cryopreservation, if a regular decreasing temperature is maintained. A cryoprotector is useful, particularly if cartilaginous cells are to be spared. The preservation temperature must be low enough to inhibit cellular activity and lytic enzymes (< –90°C).

Freeze-dried/Lyophilised Allografts

Lyophilisation used alone is no more sterilising than cryopreservation and requires the same strict rules about the selection of donors, as well as a strict asepsis procedure when taking the graft. Lyophilisation increases the fragility of grafts.

Irradiated Allografts

Irradiation in combination with lyophilisation has been used since 1958 to prepare bone allografts. Irradiation of 2.5 megarad destroys cells, bacteria and yeast, but not viruses and prions, and causes the grafts to become fragile. Grafts must be irradiated before deep-freezing. This procedure is rarely used nowadays.

Chemically Sterilised Allografts

Agents such as methiolate and propriolactone are no longer used because of their toxicity. Small grafts must be used to ensure reliable penetration and gas extraction. Chemical sterilisation is usually associated with lyophilisation, which helps gas extraction and avoids the damage caused by contact with the non-waterproof packaging of the graft.

Heat Sterilisation

Few people use this method nowadays. The allografts are biomechanically and biologically denatured by heat and their incorporation is altered. On the other hand, experimental reimplantation of autografts after an autoclave session seems to be successful. Interesting clinical results have been reported in humans using this method.

Decalcified and Deproteinised Grafts

These methods deliberately denature grafts in order to improve their incorporation. Decalcification makes osteoinduction easier. Bone resistance is damaged. As deproteinisation makes grafts fragile, it is mainly used during the preparation of xenografts.

Specific Surgical Procedures

Resection Arthrodesis of the Knee

Resection arthrodesis of the knee is one of the resection and reconstruction processes used for tumours of the lower extremity of the femur or the upper extremity of the tibia. In France, it is known as Juvara's procedure, in Italy, Putti Juvara's procedure and in Anglo-Saxon countries, the merle d'Aubigné procedure. It is used less frequently nowadays (procedures such as massive prosthesis are more common), but it remains the oldest known procedure, and the only method used before 1965. It is a two-step procedure:

- Excision of the tumour by segmentary resection of the distal parts of the femur or of the proximal parts of the tibia, or both, and in some cases a single-block arthrectomy
- Bone reconstruction, aiming at reconstructing a long femoro-tibia shaft fixed by a long centro-medullar nail.

Massive Prosthesis

Reconstruction using a massive prosthesis must be considered whenever resection of a bone segment is required because of a malignant or benign but aggressive tumour. This technique allows bone sparing and maintains satisfactory mobility:

- In tumours of the lower extremity of the femur, the carcinological excision must spare enough muscle to allow the knee to move and to stabilise it. This can be done by preserving the straight muscle of the thigh, rectus femoris and the medial great, vastus medians and vastus lateralis, which is usually possible
- In tumours of the upper extremity of the tibia, the patellar tendon, different reinsertion techniques (head of fibula, lambeau de jumeau, allografts) widen the indications for prostheses

- In tumours reaching the joint cavity, the indication is less obvious and depends on the quality of the extensor system left after a single-block arthrectomy
- In tumours of the upper extremity of the femur or of the acetabulum, a total prosthesis with an antiluxation ring covering as much of the glutens maxims as possible must be set to avoid instability.

Age is not a factor for teenagers or young adults. With a young child, sterilisation of the two metaphyses may be considered a contraindication, but the alternative resection arthrodesis procedure has similar effects on growth.

Treatment of Spinal Metastases

Radiotherapy and chemotherapy are the basic elements of treatment of spinal metastases, but surgery has very precise indications. Three complications require surgical treatment:

- Neurological complications with recent medullary or radicular compression
- Mechanical complications with destabilisation of the vertebrae
- Metastasis-related pain unrelievable by drugs, linked to bone fragility with microfractures.

In all these cases the aim is always stabilisation and often decompression. The posterior approach is much more efficient than the anterior approach. This procedure is quicker and less aggressive than thoracotomy or a surgical section of the loins. This posterior approach enables wide exploration and a wide decompression if needed. It allows an extensive laminectomy if required and peeling of an epidural tumour streak. At the cervical level, osteosynthesis is carried out using posterior plates, with screws set in vertebral pedicles.

Complementary Procedures

A posterolateral bone graft can be performed in some cases. It is justified if patients have a long life expectancy, as in those with bone metastases from breast, thyroid or prostate cancer. It is not normally performed in other cases. Consolidation of the graft is not inhibited by radiotherapy of less than 45 Gy, if required. Postoperative immobilisation is always advised if the patient has no medullary damage: a minerva plaster, a jacket for the upper cervical spine, a simple collar for the lower cervical spine and a three-point corset for the dorsal and lumbar spine (a chin holder attached to a three-point corset may be necessary for the upper dorsal spine). The patient must stay immobilised for 3 months. In cases of neurological medullary damage, a corset should be avoided because pressure sores are likely to develop.

Part 1

Histology and Experimental Study

1 Pathology of Bone Metastatic Tumours

L. Garbe-Galanti

The skeleton is the most common site of cancerous metastasis, after the lungs and liver. Metastases are four times more frequent than primary malignant tumours (Jaffé, 1958; Ewing, 1928). They occur more frequently than is generally supposed because there are not always clinical or radiological signs. Systematic research using iliac crest biopsies and studies on autopsies in large series have proved that the frequency of bone metastases is significant (50–60% among cancerous patients) (Abrams et al, 1950; Berretoni and Carter, 1986).

The metastatic lesions occur in the 5 years following treatment of the original tumour, but may also be observed after this time. The primary tumour is clinically silent in about one-third of cases and it may remain occult for a long time (only 50% of metastasis) (Simon and Bartucci, 1986; Clain, 1965). The axial bones, such as the vertebral column, skull and pelvis, represent the more frequent sites. Carcinomas of the breast, prostate, thyroid, kidney and lung constitute the great majority of bone metastases.

1.1 Techniques and Choice of Bone Sample

Indications for bone samples vary according to the clinical story. There are three types of specimen:

- Biopsies of bone marrow
- Punctures
- Surgical biopsies.

Biopsies of bone marrow are made at the level of the iliac crest after local anaesthesia. One or several samples may be obtained for cytological and histological examination. The results are very significant and more than 50% of metastasis are detected (Wassel and Cywiner-Golenzer, 1979).

Punctures are made with needles or trocars, under scanner supervision, at the vertebral level.

Surgical biopsies should be fixed in formalin, completely decalcified (except the very osteolytic metastases) and stained with hemalun-eosin-safran. For cytological examination, the sample should be fixed in alcohol-ether or cyto-spray and stained with May-Grumwald-Giemsa PAS.

1.2 Macroscopic Study

1.2.1 Localisation of Skeletal Metastasis

The involvement of the vertebral column (Fig. 1.1) has been described by Abelanet (1990). Metastases of one or several vertebrae may compress the spinal column. The metastases affect the body, pedicle or apophysis, with lysis of the bone, and are characterised by whitish spots within the red marrow. More rarely, the vertebrae are hard and have an ivory-like appearance.

The pelvis is a frequent localisation for osteolytic metastasis and spontaneous fractures. There may be a large diffusion of tumour cells within the iliac crests. Prostatic carcinoma often metastasises to the sacrum.

The skull, particularly the top, is a site for some metastases.

The sternum, ribs (Fig. 1.2) and clavicles are often very osteolytic and are preferential sites for carcinoma of the lungs.

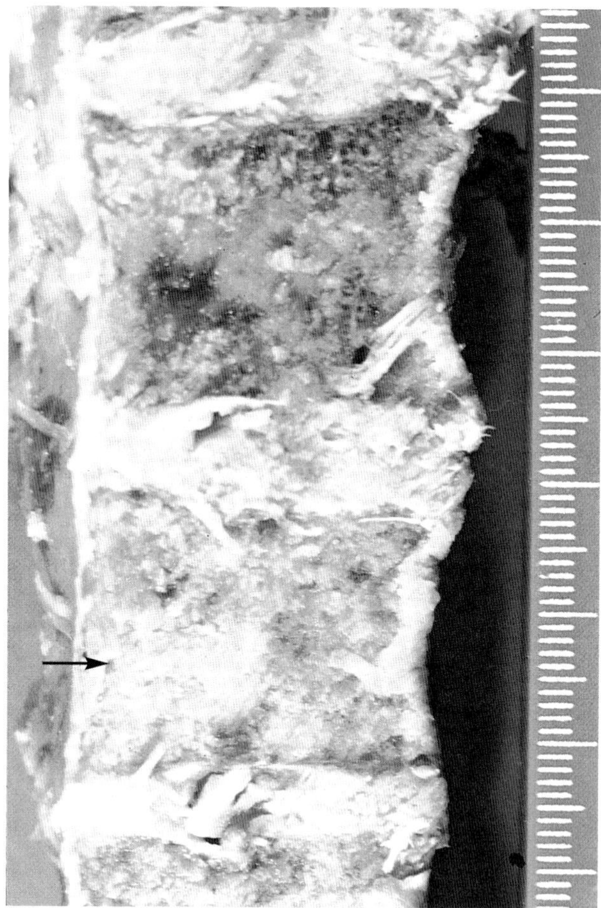

Figure 1.1 Sagittal section of two lumbar vertebrae showing whitish and irregular cancerous spots (*arrow*) (adenocarcinoma of breast)

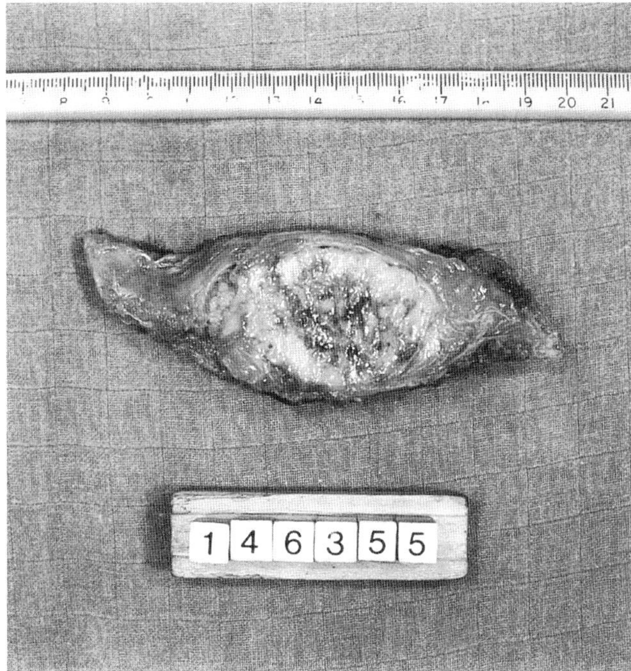

Figure 1.2 Osteolytic metastasis of a rib (squamous cell carcinoma of lung)

In the limbs, metastases are either large and single (Fig. 1.3) or small and numerous. They are often seen in the metaphysis and epiphysis of long bones, especially the femur. Distal bones are unusual sites for metastasis, but the metacarpus and metatarsus are more often involved than the phalanges (Fechner and Mills, 1993).

1.2.2 Metastatic Types

There are several types of metastases:

- Bone marrow
- Osteolytic
- Osteoblastic
- Mixed.

In bone marrow metastasis, the architecture of the bone and the X-ray are normal because the metastasis is very often small and tumour cells spread only in the marrow without destruction of bone. The diagnosis will be apparent only on histological examination.

Osteolytic metastases are frequent and often lead to spontaneous fractures. The tumour nodules are necrotic and whitish; they more or less destroy the spongy

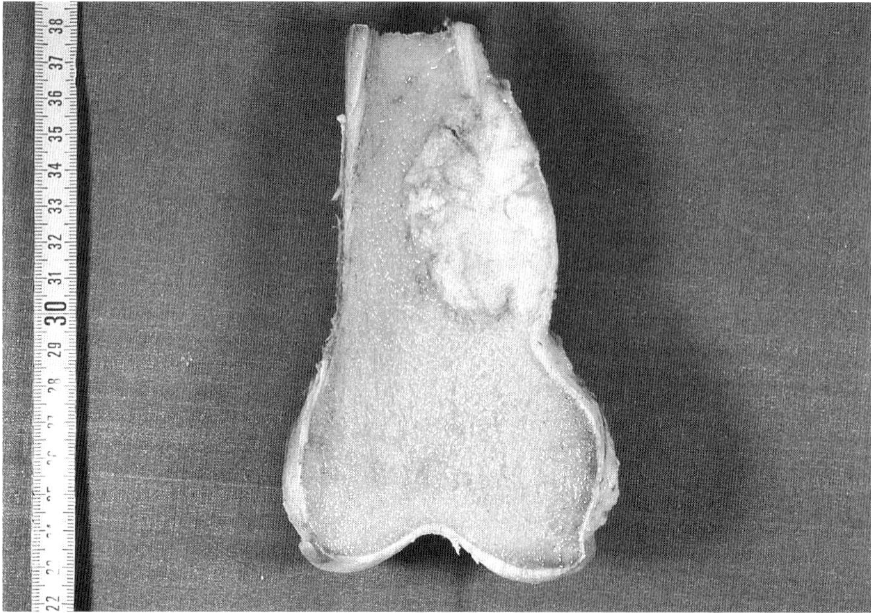

Figure 1.3 Sagittal section of a femur with a large metastasis in the metaphysis. The macroscopic feature looks like a primary tumour of bone (carcinoma of bladder)

and cortical bone (Figs 1.4, 1.5). Carcinomas of the thyroid, kidney, gastro-intestinal tract and lungs lead to large osteolytic metastases.

Osteoblastic metastases result from carcinomas of the breast and prostate in particular (Meyer, 1957). They do not often lead to spontaneous fractures, as the bones are very hard and yellow, like ivory. These metastases are more often diffuse and localised in the axial skeleton.

In mixed metastases, necrosis and osteoblastic formations are associated (Fig. 1.6). Carcinoma of the breast is often the cause of these diffused metastases.

1.3 Histological Study

1.3.1 Clinical Situations

It is important that the pathologist is aware of the clinical situation.

If the primary tumour is known and metastasis has occurred in the 3–5 years following therapy, it is important to ensure that it is a metastasis. The histological features are generally easy to diagnose even if the lesion appears small or undifferentiated in relation to the primary tumour.

If the primary tumour is clinically silent and the metastasis suggests an unknown malignant tumour, histological examination of the metastasis will allow orientation or clarification of the starting point. This is easier when the bone tumour exactly reproduces the original lesion, for example, carcinomas of the kidney (Fig. 1.7), thyroid, oat-cell carcinoma of the lung, pigmented melanoma, malignant lymphoma, sometimes carcinomas of the breast (Fig. 1.8) and colon, and adenoid cystic

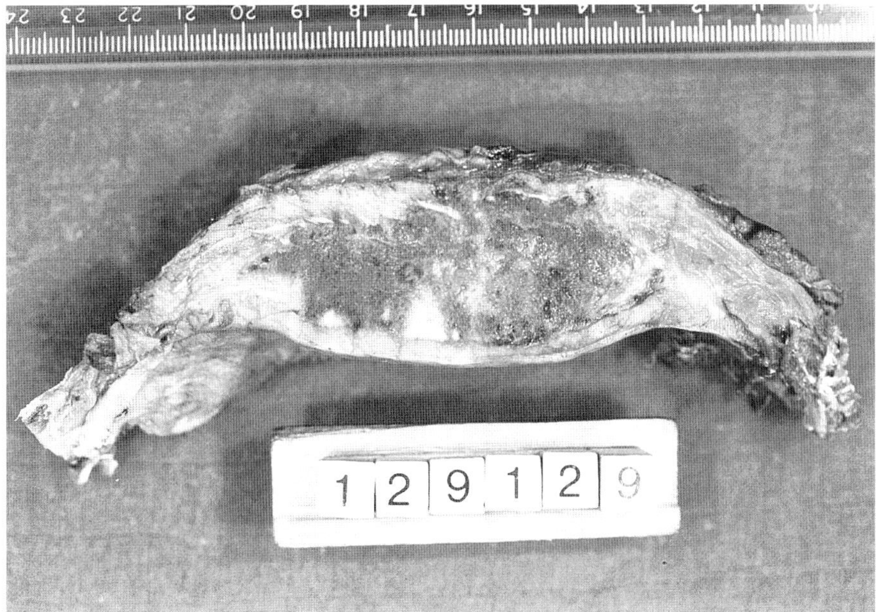

Figure 1.4 Voluminous and necrotic tumour nodule in a rib (adenocarcinoma of lung)

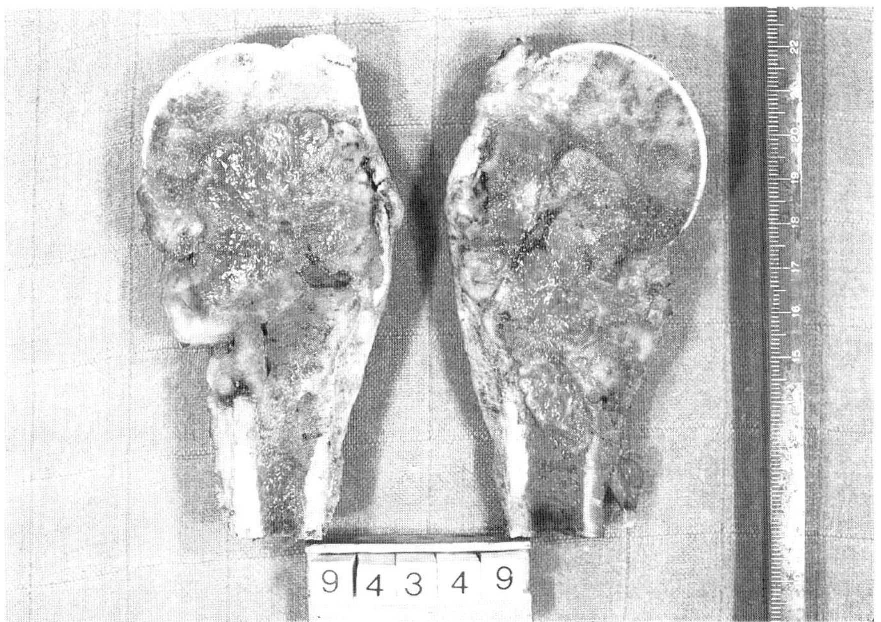

Figure 1.5 Osteolytic and necrotic metastasis in epiphysis of a humerus (hypernephroma)

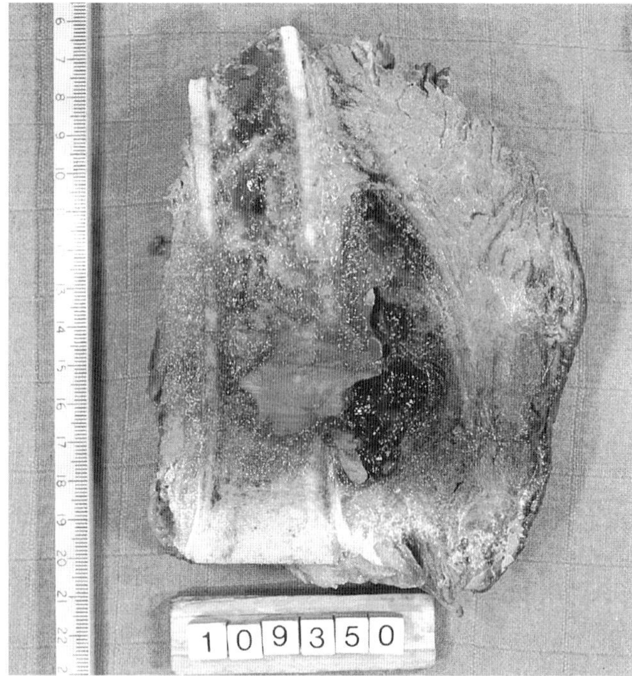

Figure 1.6 Mixed metastasis of a humerus with osteolytic necrotic and osteoblastic features (adenocarcinoma of liver)

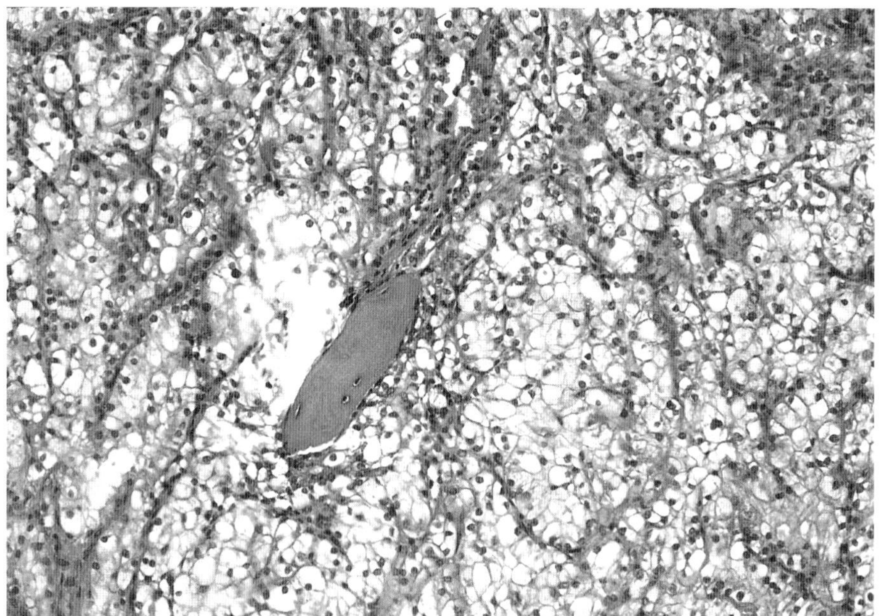

Figure 1.7 Clear and vegetal cells surrounding bone tissue (adenocarcinoma of kidney) (original magnification x250)

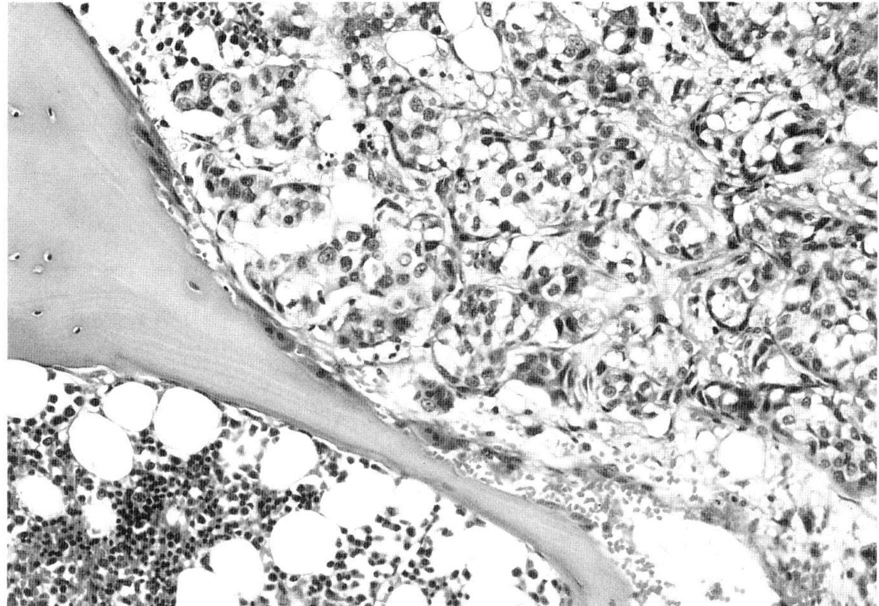

Figure 1.8 Nests of tumour cells in contact with normal marrow (adenocarcinoma of breast) (original magnification x250)

carcinoma (Fig. 1.9). It is more difficult when the metastasis is undifferentiated, with few cells trapped in a fibrosing stromal reaction. The pathologist will be able to identify a tumour type, such as squamous cell carcinoma or adenocarcinoma with mucoid secretion (Fig. 1.10), but the primary tumour will not be localised with certainty and complementary investigations will be required to find it.

Metastasis in children presents some unique features. Ewing's sarcomas, neuroblastomas and osteosarcomas (Fig. 1.11) often lead to bone metastasis, but medulloblastomas and hypernephromas do so less often.

1.3.2 Morphology of Bone Metastasis

Bone metastases either reproduce the primary tumour or appear more or less undifferentiated. Morphological appearances vary according to whether the metastasis is osteolytic or osteoblastic.

In osteolytic metastasis, there are two mechanisms for bone destruction:

- Increased osteoclastic activity by the action of cellular factors; osteoclasts are numerous and voluminous (Fig. 1.12) with dense fibrosis (Aoki et al, 1988)
- Circulatory problems at the level of certain bones (vertebrae): the vascularisation is altered by strong mechanical pressures leading to a progressive bone melting with ischaemic necrosis.

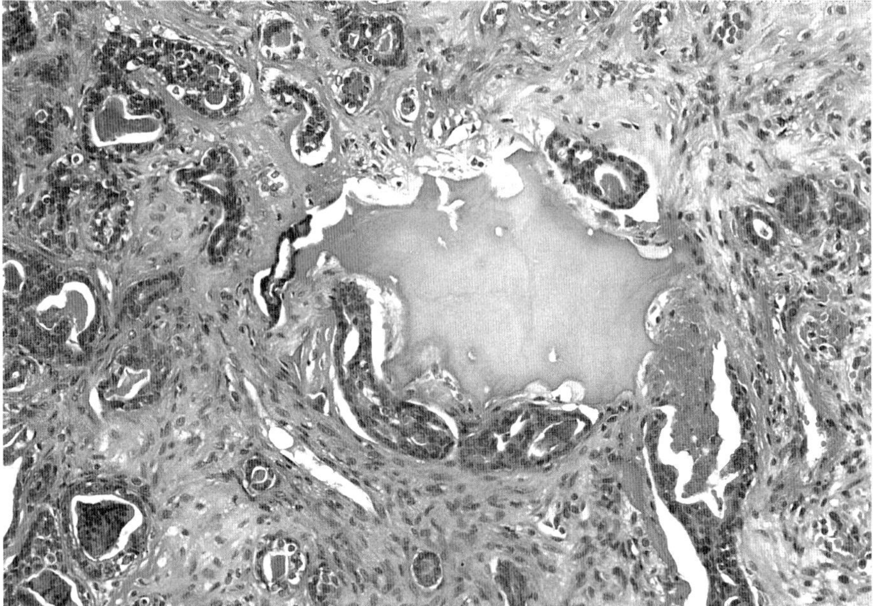

Figure 1.9 Tubular formations with acidophilic substance in the lumen and hyalin stroma (adenoid cystic carcinoma) (original magnification x100)

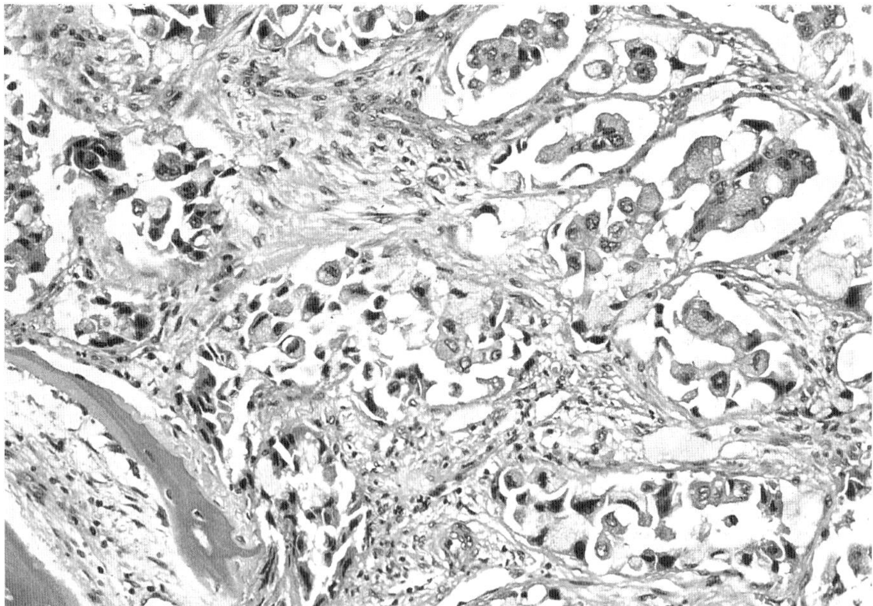

Figure 1.10 Tumour secreting cells with abundant mucinous substance in the cytoplasm (adenocarcinoma of gastrointestinal tract) (original magnification x250)

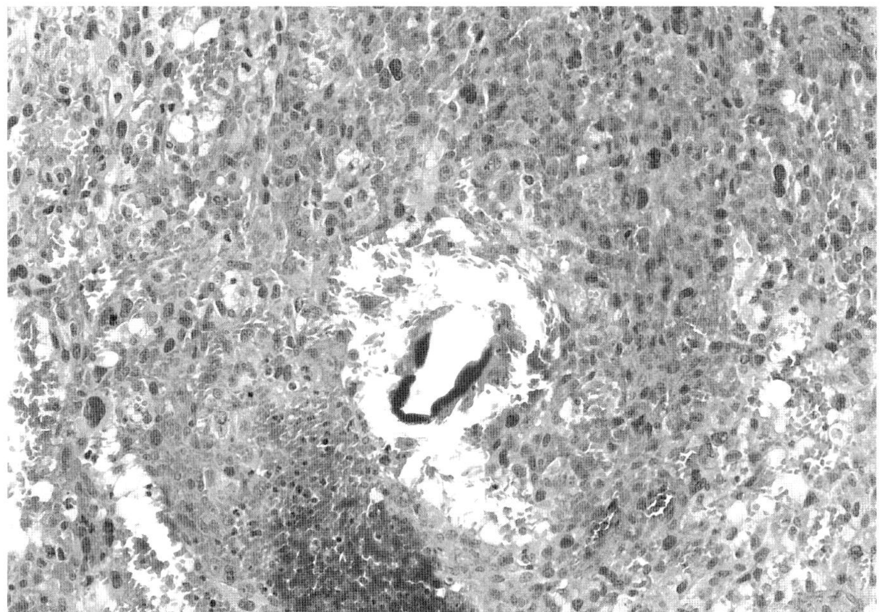

Figure 1.11 Atypical tumour cells of osteosarcoma (original magnification x100)

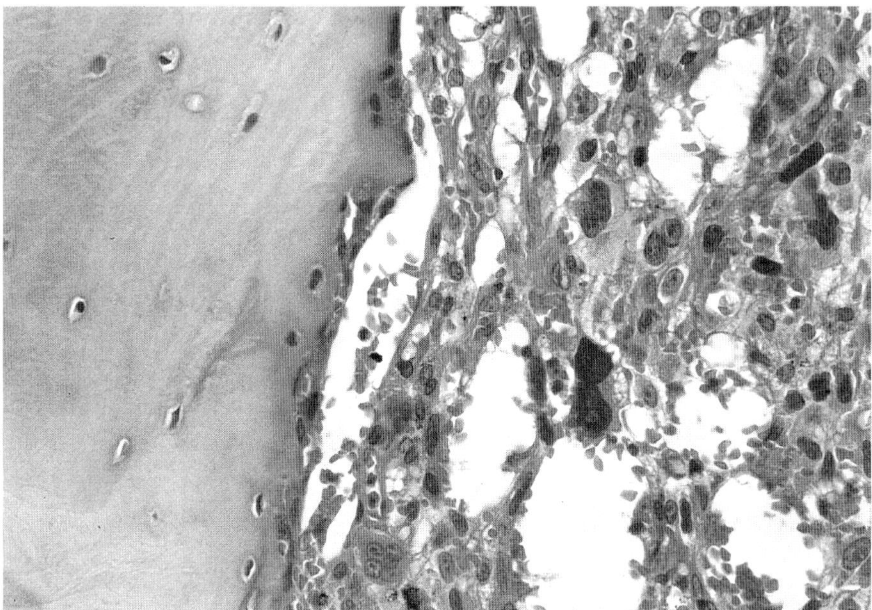

Figure 1.12 Voluminous and numerous osteoclasts in contact with bone (hypernephroma) (original magnification x400)

In osteoblastic metastasis, tumour cells cause new ossification by three mechanisms:

- Metaplasia within the fibrous cancerous stroma
- Development of osteoid immature tissue perpendicular to residual bone
- Reaction of the periosteum with anarchical new bone tissue perpendicular to the pre-existing bone axis.

In bone marrow metastasis (Roeckel, 1974), tumour cells arrive at the sinus of the bone marrow. They may be difficult to examine within a dense fibrosis. Sometimes, however, tumour cells are voluminous and destroy the blood tissue.

1.3.3 Diagnostic Problems and Immunohistochemistry

In some metastases, the morphology is very difficult to identify. A bone metastasis comprised only of round undifferentiated cells may be a metastasis or a primary tumour; it may be a neuroblastoma, Ewing's sarcoma, round-cell osteosarcoma or malignant lymphoma. In addition, a spindle-cell tumour may derive from a pseudosarcomatous carcinoma (kidney) or an original or secondary sarcoma.

Immunohistochemistry has been used for several years to specify the diagnosis (Le Doussal and Amouroux, 1997). Several types of antibody may be used:

- Epithelial cell antibodies (cytokeratins, epithelial membrane antigen) to identify the carcinomatous nature of the metastasis
- Connective and histiocytic cell antibodies (vimentin, actin, CD 68) to identify a sarcomatous process
- Lymphoid cell antibodies (CD 45, CD 3, L26) to recognise a malignant lymphoma.
- Endothelial cell antibodies necessary for the diagnosis of vascular tumours (factor VIII, BNH9, CD 34).

All these antibodies are targeted against the usual components of the tissues and specific antibodies of organs. There are too many to mention them all here. Which antibody to use depends on the particular clinical and morphological situation. In the future, more specific antibodies will lead to a better outcome. The routine use of growth and cellular proliferation factors and resistance factors to chemotherapy will increase the accuracy of diagnosis of bone metastasis when the primary tumour is clinically silent.

1.4 Mechanisms of Development of Bone Metastasis

The development of tumour cells within the bone tissue depends on several factors (Berretoni and Carter, 1986), which lead to the appearance of osteolytic or osteoblastic metastases.

1.4.1 Function of Cellular Factors

Tumour cells secrete chemotactic substances, which increase the action of osteoclasts (osteolytic metastasis) (Galasko, 1982; Orr et al, 1978) or stimulate osteoblasts (osteoblastic metastasis). Moreover, receptors on the surface of tumour cells (Berretoni and Carter, 1986) may be responsible for their progress towards the bone marrow and their adhesion to the walls of the medullary sinus.

1.4.2 Function of the Osseous Vascular Network

Arteries and veins may bring tumour cells from the primary tumour to the bone (Ewing, 1928; Borg et al, 1993). The arterial circulation ends in the capillaries of the haematopoietic tissue, especially in the metaphysis and epiphysis of long bones. At this level, the slower circulation favours the introduction of tumour cells. In the venous network, tumour cells circulate in the vertebral system, which forms an anastomosis between the vertebral and caval venous systems from the pelvis to the skull (frequent axial metastasis) (Batson, 1942). However, tumour cells have typical and specific features favouring their penetration into the vascular walls, because the presence of tumour cells in a biopsy does not always lead to the development of bone metastasis in the future.

1.5 Summary

Bone metastases are very frequent but probably underestimated, as shown by studies on iliac crest biopsies. They may be indicative of a clinically silent tumour. The diagnosis is based on biopsies of bone marrow, needle puncture of suspicious zones or surgical biopsies. The spine, skull and pelvis are the most common sites, but the ribs and the epiphysis and metaphysis of long bones may also be affected. Metastases in the distal bones are rare, but are more likely to affect the metatarsal and metacarpal bones than the phalanges. Some tumours (breast, prostate, thyroid, kidney and lung) have specific affinities for the bone tissue.

Bone metastases may occur only in the marrow, they may cause widespread destruction of the bone, or they may lead to an osteoblastic appearance. Histologically, the diagnosis is easy if the primary tumour is known, but difficult when the original cancer is silent. In some cases, the pathologist will be able to specify the starting point with certainty. More often, it will only be possible to suggest a diagnosis without confirmation of the origin, unless the metastasis is very differentiated and reproduces the primary tumour (hypernephroma, oat-cell carcinoma of lung, adenocarcinoma of thyroid). In these circumstances, immunohistochemistry helps to specify the diagnosis. The mechanisms of metastatic growth involve cellular chemotactic factors and connections with the caval venous system at the vertebral level, in the vascular bone network.

References

Abelanet R (1990) Métastases osseuses: anatomie pathologique. In: Tomeno B, Forest M (eds) Les tumeurs osseuses de l'appareil locomoteur. Laboratoires Unicet, pp 1–18.

Abrams HC, Spiro R, Goldstein N (1950) Metastases in carcinoma: analysis of 1000 autopsied cases. Cancer 3:74–85.

Aoki J, Yamamoto I, Shigeno C et al (1988) Osteoclast mediated osteolysis in bone metastasis from renal cell carcinoma. Cancer 62:98–144.

Batson OV (1942) The function of the vertebral veins in metastatic processes. Ann Intern Med 16:38–45.
Berretoni BA, Carter JR (1986) Mechanisms of cancer metastasis to bone. J Bone Joints Surg 68A:308–312.
Borg SA, Rubin P, Dewys WD (1993) Metastases and disseminated disease. In: Rubin P (ed) Clinical oncology for medical students and physicians. A multidisciplinary approach, 6th edn. American Cancer Society, New York, pp 498–499.
Clain A (1965) Secondary malignant disease of bone. Br J Cancer 19:15–29.
Ewing J (1928) Metastasis in neoplastic disease. A textbook on tumors. Saunders, Philadelphia, pp 77–89
Fechner RE, Mills SE (1993) Tumors of the bones and joints. AFIP, Washington.
Galasko CSB (1982) Mechanisms of lytic and blastic metastatic disease of bone. Clin Orthop 160–207.
Jaffe HL (1958) Tumors and tumorous conditions of the bones and joints. Lea and Febiger, Philadelphia.
Le Doussal V, Amouroux J (1997) Métastases osseuses: apport de l'anatomie pathologique. In: Cancers secondaires des os. Expansion Scientifique Franc[,]aise, pp 71–80.
Meyer PC (1957) A statistical and histological survey of metastatic carcinoma of the skeleton. Br J Cancer 12:109–568.
Orr FW, Varani J, Ward PA (1978) Characteristics of the chemotactic response of neoplastic cells to a factor derived from fifth component of complement. Am J Pathol 93:405–422.
Roeckel LE (1974) Diagnosis of metastatic carcinoma by bone marrow biopsy versus bone marrow aspiration. Ann Clin Lab Sci 4:193–197.
Simon MA, Bartucci EJ (1986) The search for the primary tumor in patients with skeletal metastasis of unknown origin. Cancer 58:1088–1095.
Wassel F, Cywiner-Golenzer CH (1979) Les métastases osseuses des cancers. Retentissement sur le tissu osseux et médullaire. Arch Anat Cytol Pathol 27:337–342.

Part 2

Identification

2 Radiographic Imaging of Skeletal Metastases

M. Panuel, Ph. Petit, F. Portier and Ch. Chagnaud

Imaging is an important clue in the diagnosis of skeletal metastases. In the imaging armamentarium, the place of conventional radiographic examination has to be defined. The radiographic appearances of skeletal metastases are related to the mechanisms of bone involvement and to the patterns of bone response. Bone metastases are usually encountered in middle-aged and elderly patients but may also occur in children. In adults, carcinomas of the lung, prostate, breast and kidney account for more than 75% of skeletal metastases; in children, neuroblastoma is the main cause.

2.1 Mechanisms of Bone Involvement

The majority of skeletal metastases are haematogeneous in origin. Two pathways exist: the arterial system and the venous system, although their relative roles are difficult to establish. However, the prominent role of the vertebral venous plexus of Batson has been clearly highlighted in metastatic spread in the ribs, spine and pelvis. Other data illustrate the role of haematogeneous dissemination: there is a concordance with the usual sites of skeletal metastases and the remaining areas of red marrow, areas that are richly vascularised. A similar observation may be made concerning cortical or subperiosteal metastases, which develop in the periosteal plexus. In the metastases arising in cancellous bone, the first step is involvement of the bone marrow, followed by an osseous involvement. Direct extension, such as in the case of Pancoast-Tobias' syndrome, lymphatic spread or intrathecal dissemination to the bone are less likely to be mechanisms of bone metastases (Resnick and Niwayama, 1995).

2.2 Osseous Response to Metastases

Implantation of tumour cells in the bone leads to several types of response: bone resorption, bone formation or mixed response.

2.2.1 Resorption

Resorption may occur by osteoclast-mediated osteolysis or by direct destruction due to the development of tumour cells (Resnick and Niwayama, 1995). The role of humoral substances such as prostaglandins, osteoclast-activating factor or other unidentified agents has been suggested (Kitazawa and Maeda, 1995). The bone destruction is usually not radiographically detectable by plain films until approximately 50% of a focal region of bone has been destroyed (Pagani and Libshitz, 1982; Resnick and Niwayama, 1995). A destructive focus will be more apparent in the cortex than in the medulla and more easily seen in bone of normal density than in osteoporotic bone (Greenfield, 1990). Destruction may involve the medulla, the cortex or both. The limits with the adjacent bone may be sharp or ill-defined, reflecting the aggressiveness of the lesion as well as the presence of reactive new bone. Bone resorption is the most common type of response and occurs in almost all types of cancer, particularly carcinoma of the breast, lung, kidney, thyroid and malignant skin tumours.

2.2.2 Bone Formation

Bone formation may accompany the development of skeletal metastases. New bone is deposited on pre-existing trabeculae and in the trabecular spaces, probably due to direct stimulation of osteoblasts by the tumour cells and their humoral agents. This new bone formation may be nodular, mottled or diffuse (Resnick and Niwayama, 1995). The most frequently seen osteoblastic metastases are from carcinoma of the prostate, but may also be encountered with bronchial carcinoid tumour or carcinoma of the nasopharynx.

2.2.3 Mixed Response

Mixed response is seen more rarely. It generally occurs in lung, breast and ovarian cancer. Individual patients respond differently to metastatic disease.

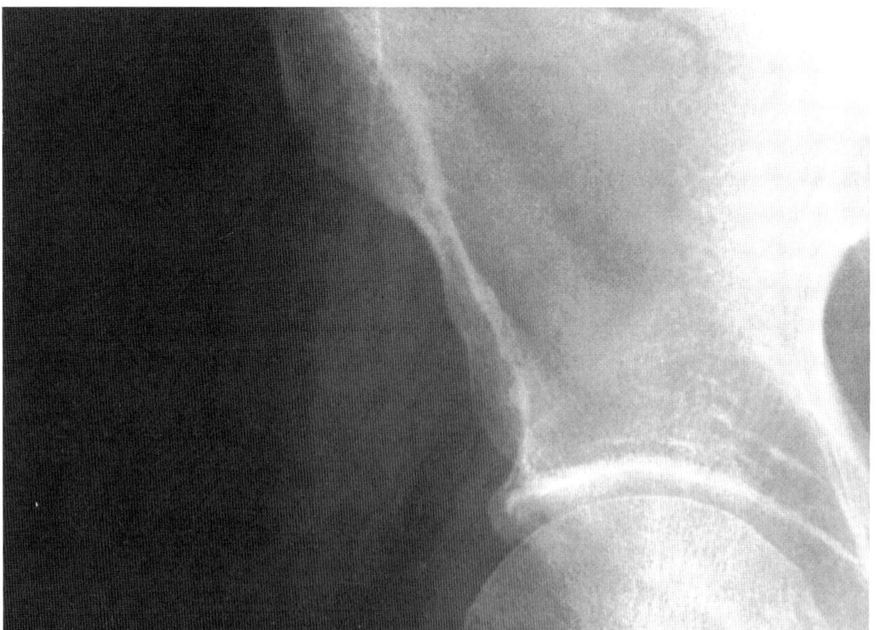

Figure 2.1 Lytic bladder carcinoma metastasis in the right ilium with a "moth-eaten" appearance

2.3 Radiographic Imaging

The radiographic patterns of skeletal metastases include alterations in bone density and structure, and are variable according to the type of bone response, the nature of the primary tumour, the age of the patient, the location and the number of metastatic foci (Resnick and Niwayama, 1995; Greenfield, 1990; Rieden, 1995).

2.3.1 Osteolytic Lesions

Osteolytic lesions are usually ill-defined and poorly marginated or may be well circumscribed, giving a "moth-eaten" or a geographic appearance respectively (Figs 2.1 and 2.2). Pathological fractures may occur on tubular bones and

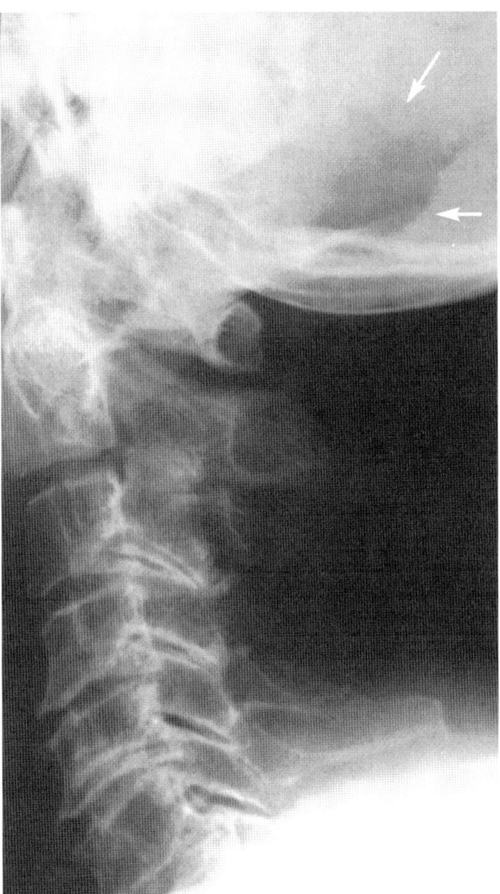

Figure 2.2 Lytic bronchogenic carcinoma metastases in the occipital bone and the spinous process of C4. The occipital metastasis has a geographic appearance

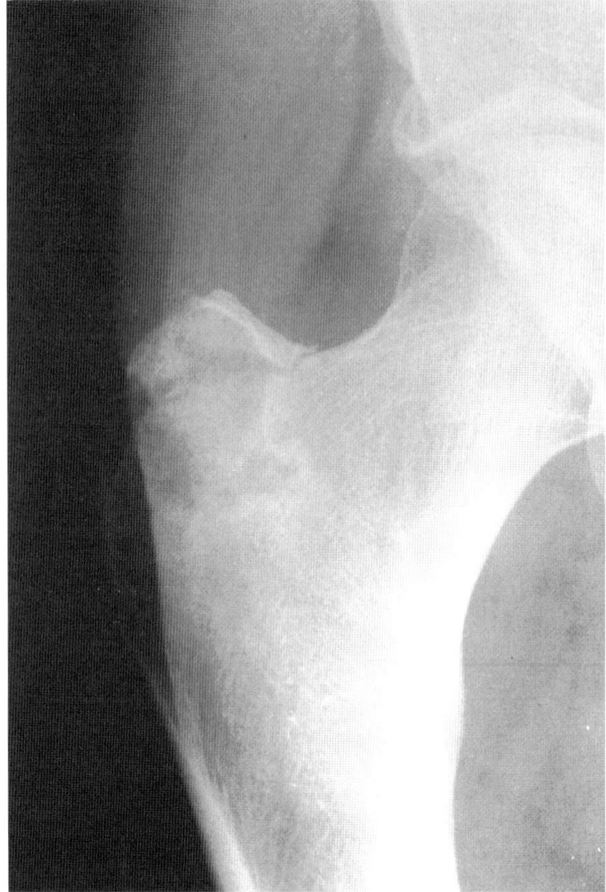

Figure 2.3 Lytic breast carcinoma metastasis in the greater trochanter with pathological fracture and sclerotic rim

vertebral bodies (Fig. 2.3). When the vertebrae are involved, particularly with vertebral collapse, the radiographic findings may suggest the metastatic origin: involvement of the upper thoracic spine (although all segments may be involved), presence of adjacent soft tissue mass, destruction of one or both pedicles (absence of one or both "eyes" of the vertebra on the antero-posterior view),

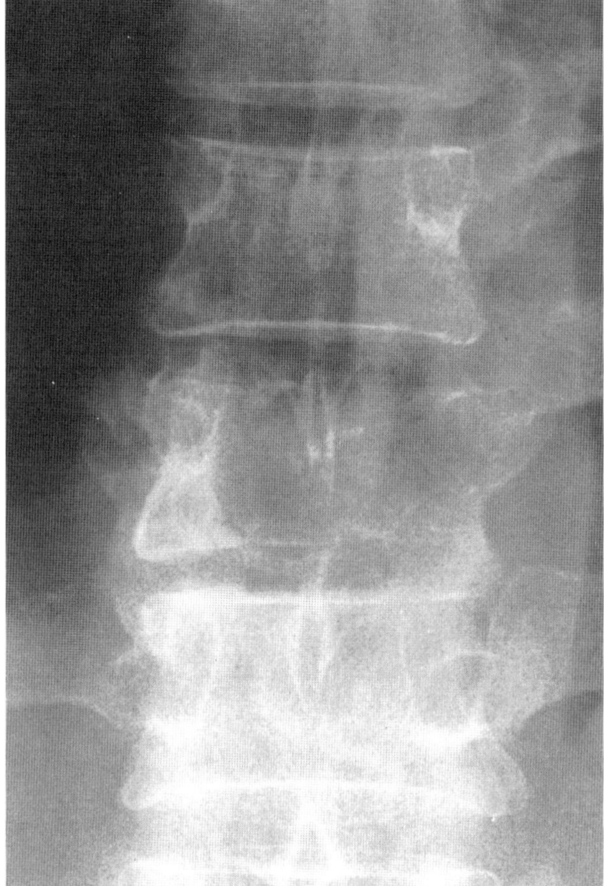

Figure 2.4 Lytic breast carcinoma metastasis of the T10 vertebra with subtle collapse, irregularities of the upper end plate, destruction of the left pedicle and soft tissue mass

angular or irregular deformity of the vertebral endplates (Fig. 2.4). As a general rule, the intervertebral spaces and joint spaces are usually preserved.

Subperiosteal or cortical metastasis, giving a "saucerisation" appearance, is uncommon, usually resulting from carcinoma of the lung or kidney ("cookie-bite sign") (Figs 2.5 and 2.6). Subperiosteal or cortical localisation accounts for less

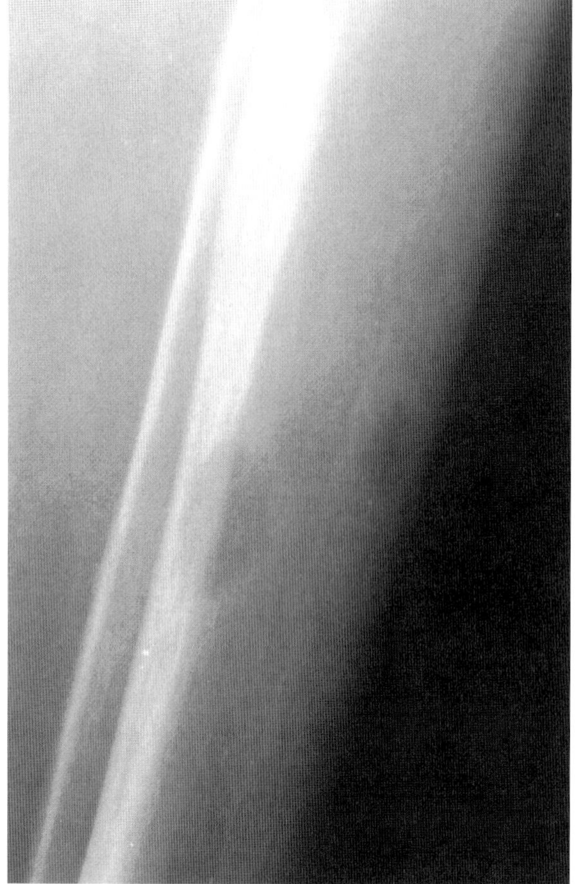

Figure 2.5 Two lytic cortical metastases of the tibia from carcinoma of the colon

than 30% of metastases of the appendicular skeleton (Coerkamp and Kroon, 1988).

2.3.2 Osteoblastic Metastases

Osteoblastic metastases appear as ill-defined areas of increased density or as a diffuse sclerosis (Figs 2.7 and 2.8). Very rarely, all the bones may be involved with uniform sclerosis (Greenfield, 1990). On the other hand, a dense vertebral body ("ivory vertebra") may be observed.

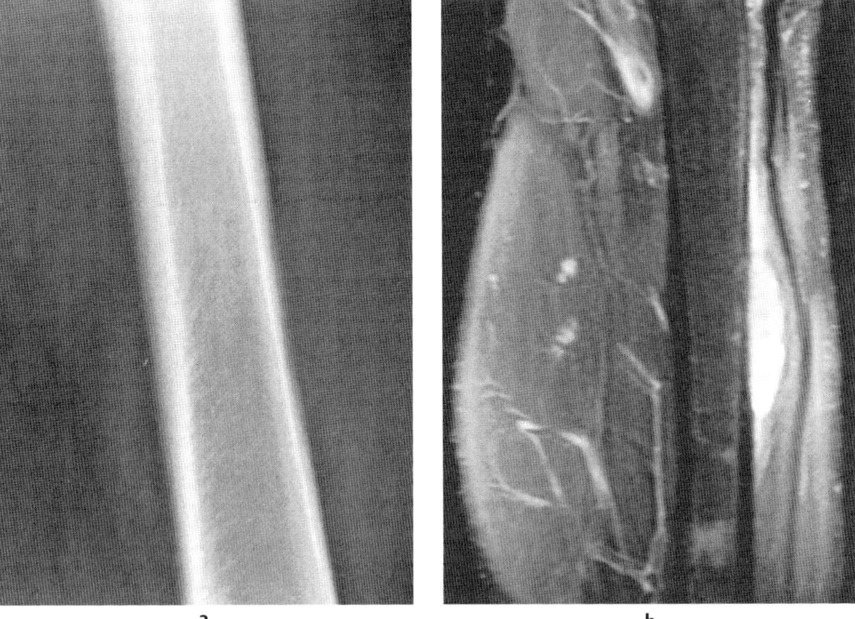

Figure 2.6 Subperiosteal metastasis of the femur from carcinoma of the lung. **a** Plain film. Subtle "cookie-bite" sign. **b** MRI, sagittal plane, T2-weighted image. Soft tissue mass accompanying the bone erosion. Courtesy of Dr Dubayle

In some instances, metastases from carcinoma of the kidney or thyroid, either osteolytic or osteoblastic, may lead to bone expansion, related to the hypervascularity of the lesion (Fig. 2.9). Periosteal reaction is uncommon, but in unusual circumstances, an exuberant periosteal reaction with bone spiculation, and sometimes bone expansion, may be observed with metastases arising from prostatic carcinoma or neuroblastoma. Unusual sites of metastases are the extremities (terminal phalanges, carpal or tarsal bones); in such cases, bronchogenic carcinoma is the main cause (Figs 2.10 and 2.11).

2.4 Role of the Radiographic Examination in the Evaluation of Skeletal Metastases

The circumstances differ according to whether the primary neoplasm is known.

In asymptomatic patients, when the neoplasm is known and the rate of skeletal metastasis is high, because of the low sensitivity of the plain radiographic examination, a conventional radiographic survey, including all parts of the skeleton, should be avoided. In such circumstances, bone scintigraphy is still the method of choice, although false-negative or false-positive bone scans may be encountered (McNeil, 1984). When bone scintigraphy is positive, plain radiographic films can

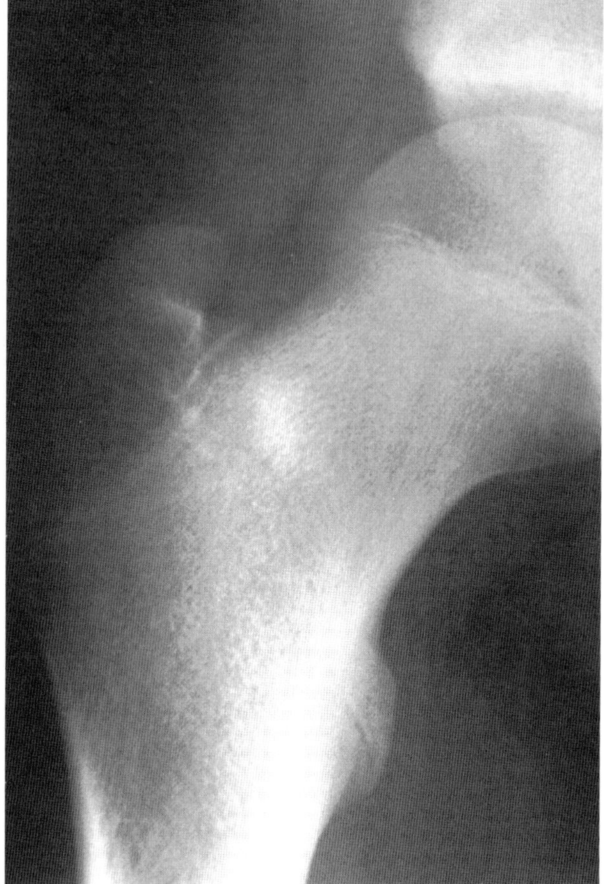

Figure 2.7 Blastic metastasis of the right femoral neck from osteosarcoma of the tibia

be confined to the foci of scintigraphic abnormality. Examination by computed tomography (CT), particularly of special areas such as pelvic bones or vertebrae, may be helpful to analyse the lesion. When the radiographic examination (conventional films and CT) of the area is normal, magnetic resonance imaging (MRI) may be indicated (Franck et al, 1990). Moreover, MRI of the spine and pelvis could be considered as a survey for bone metastases because of its high sensitivity (Neumann et al, 1995).

When the neoplasm is known and when local symptoms or pain occur, the first method of evaluation is the plain radiographic examination. On the appendicular skeleton, it can more or less assess the risk of a pending fracture, which is likely if more than 50% of the cortex is destroyed (Fiedler, 1981). When the plain films

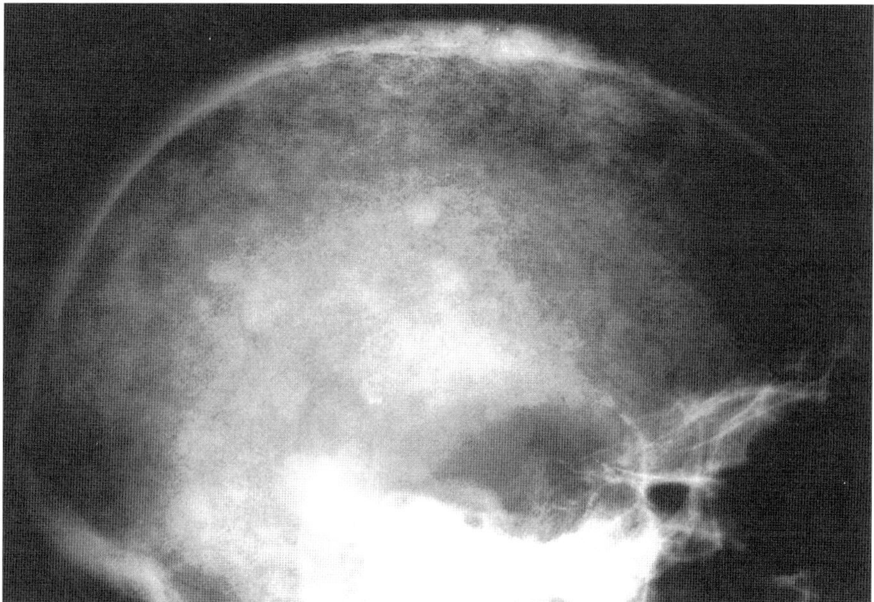

Figure 2.8 Multiple blastic metastases of the cranial vault arising from carcinoma of the prostate. The involvement of the skull bones is unusual in carcinoma of the prostate

are normal or in the presence of spinal symptoms such as cord or root nerve compression, MRI has to be performed (Soderlund, 1996).

When the primary neoplasm is unknown, a skeletal metastasis is usually discovered in the patient with local symptoms. Here again, plain films are the first step. When the patient has solitary or multiple bone abnormalities, differential diagnosis between metastases, primary bone tumour, haematological disorders, osteomyelitis or other entities may be difficult. Although the radiographic characteristics may help to differentiate between these entities, a biopsy is often needed to confirm the nature of the lesion.

The follow-up of skeletal metastases during the course of tumour therapy may be made by conventional radiography (Galasko, 1995). Healing response of an osteolytic or mixed lesion will appear as a sclerotic rim, then a progressive sclerosis; lack of response will appear as the development of osteolysis and/or the occurrence of other lesions. Metastases that are initially blastic, even in cases with a positive response, may remain osteosclerotic or disappear; on the other hand, an increase in size or development of lytic changes indicates failure of the treatment (Pagani and Libshitz, 1982). In some cases, the radiographic changes are not obvious and accurate evaluation of the response cannot be made radiographically.

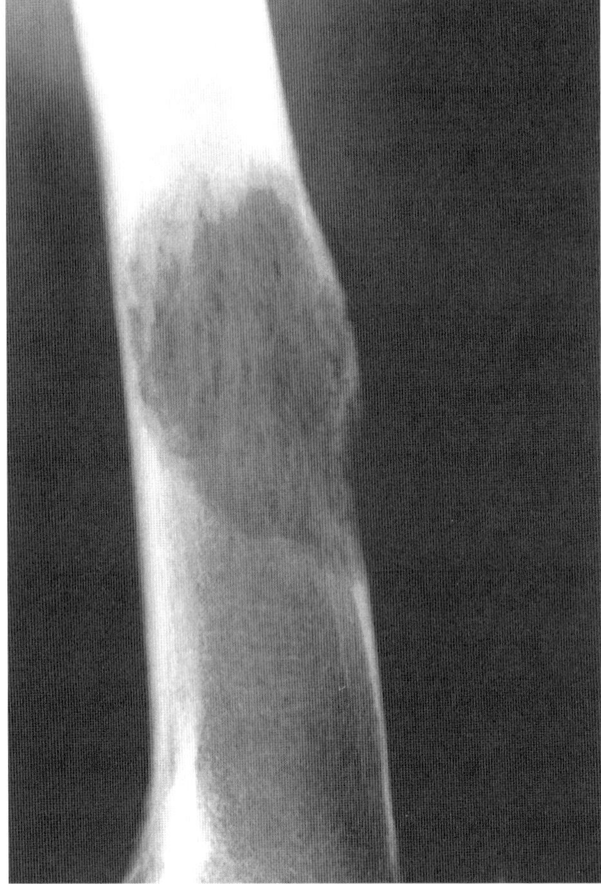

Figure 2.9 Expansile and mixed metastasis of the femur arising from carcinoma of the kidney

2.5 Summary

Skeletal metastases may appear radiographically as osteolytic, osteoblastic or mixed lesions. As a general rule, the radiographic appearance of a skeletal metastasis does not necessarily indicate the primary lesion. However, in some clinical instances, the radiographic findings may be very evocative.

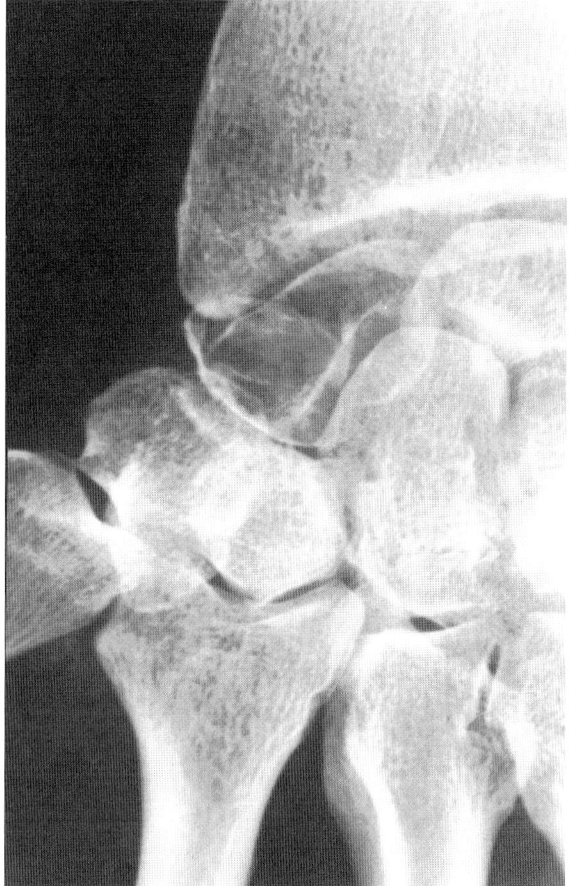

Figure 2.10 Lytic metastasis of the scaphoid bone from carcinoma of the lung with a pathological fracture

Due to the distribution of the red marrow, the axial skeleton is predominantly involved, but metastases of the appendicular skeleton may be observed.

The conventional radiographic examination has a low sensitivity in detecting metastases. Bone scintigraphy is still the method of choice for screening these metastases. Nevertheless, plain films may be very useful in the diagnosis and evaluation of the risk of a pathological fracture in the case of local symptoms in a patient with a known or unknown primary neoplasm. Assessment of the response to therapy with conventional radiography is sometimes inaccurate.

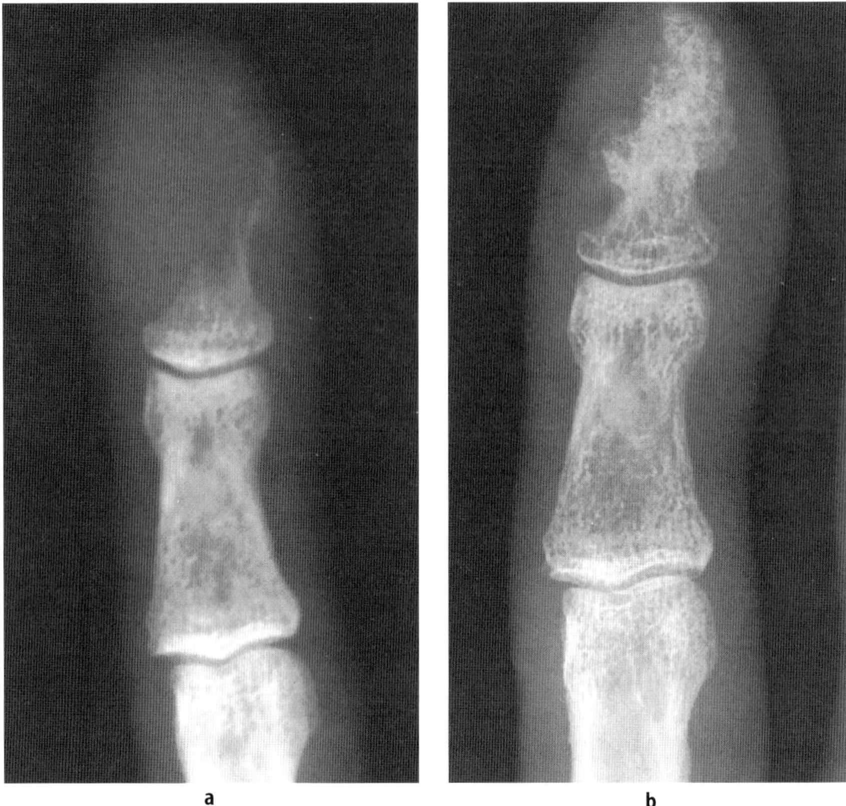

Figure 2.11 **a** Lytic metastatic lesion from carcinoma of the lung of the terminal phalanx of a finger with soft tissue enlargement. **b** Same lesion after radiation and chemotherapy. Decrease of the soft tissue mass and partial bone reconstruction, indicating a temporary response to the treatment

References

Coerkamp EG, Kroon HM (1988) Cortical bone metastases. Radiology 169:525–529.

Fiedler M (1981) Incidence of fracture through metastases in long bones. Acta Orthopedica 52:623–628.

Franck JA, Ling A, Patronas NJ et al. (1990) Detection of malignant bone tumours: MR imaging vs scintigraphy. Am J Roentgenol 155:1043–1048.

Galasko CS (1995) Diagnosis of skeletal metastases and assessment of response to treatment. Clin Orthoped 312:64–75.

Greenfield GB (1990) Cardinal roentgen features. In: Greenfield GB (ed) Radiology of bone diseases. JB Lippincott, Philadelphia, pp 405–578.

Kitazawa S, Maeda S (1995) Development of skeletal metastases. Clin Orthoped 312:45–50

McNeil BJ (1984) Value of bone scanning in neoplastic disease. Semin Nuclear Med 14:277–286.

Neumann K, Hosten N, Venz S (1995) Screening for skeletal metastases of the spine and pelvis: gradient-echo opposed-phase MRI compared with bone scintigraphy. Eur Radiol 5–3:276–284.

Pagani JJ, Libshitz HI (1982) Imaging bone metastases. Radiol Clin North Amer 20:545–560.

Resnick D, Niwayama G (1995) Skeletal metastases. In: Resnick D (ed) Diagnosis of bone and joint disorders. WB Saunders, Philadelphia, pp 3991–4064.

Rieden K (1995) Conventional imaging and computerized tomography in diagnosis of skeletal metastases. Radiologe 35:15–20.

Soderlund V (1996) Radiological diagnosis of skeletal metastases. Eur Radiol 6:587–595.

Part 3

Medical Treatment

3 Chemotherapy

F. Duffaud, P. Fumoleau and R. Favre

The incidence of bone metastases varies considerably from one tumour to another. They are especially common from carcinomas arising in the breast (73%), prostate (68%) and lung (36%). These three tumours alone account for 80% of patients with bone metastases (Coleman, 1994; Nielsen et al, 1991). Most other primary tumours can metastasise to bone, including thyroid, kidney, endometrium, cervix, bladder and gastrointestinal tract cancers, but these sites account for less than 20% of patients with bone metastases (Nielsen et al, 1991).

Treatment of bone metastases is primarily palliative. The aims of treatment are to relieve pain, to prevent development of pathological fractures, to improve mobility and function and, if possible, to prolong survival. A multidisciplinary approach is usually required to obtain the best results, involving medical oncologists, radiotherapists, surgeons, nurses and specialists in pain control. The therapeutic approach includes both local treatment (surgery and/or radiotherapy) and systemic treatment. This chapter focuses on chemotherapy in palliating patients with bone metastases. The indications for this treatment modality will depend on the primary tumour type.

In general, metastatic bone disease is an incurable condition. Nevertheless, chemotherapy is usually curative for testicular germ cell tumours, lymphoma (usually high-grade non-Hodgkin's lymphoma and Hodgkin's lymphoma) and acute lymphoblastic leukaemia (Coleman, 1994). Chemotherapy is demonstrably effective in the treatment of bone metastases in malignancies such as breast cancer and SCLC (Nielsen et al, 1991). Table 3.1 indicates the sensitivity of different cancers to chemotherapy. The discussion concentrates on chemotherapy

Table 3.1. Chemosensitivity of different tumours (modified from Marty, 1994)

Curable with chemotherapy	Major chemosensitivity response (R) >60%	Relative chemosensitivity 40%–60%	Moderate chemosensitivity 40%–20%	Low chemosensitivity R<20%
Lymphoma (non-Hodgkin's) Hodgkin's lymphoma Seminoma Embryonal carcinoma LAL, MLA*	Small-cell lung cancer Breast cancer	Ovarian cancer Head and neck cancer Gastric cancer Cervical cancer Sarcomas	Oesophagus cancer Colon cancer Non-small-cell lung cancer Bladder cancer	Renal cancer Melanoma Liver cancer Prostate cancer?

* Lymphoblastic acute leukaemia; Myeloblastic acute leukaemia

of tumours such as breast, lung, prostate and renal cancer. The literature on chemotherapy is difficult to evaluate.

3.1 Problems of Response Assessment in Skeletal Metastases

Response rates of osseous metastases to chemotherapy are often reported to be low as a consequence of difficulties in objective assessment. In 1977, on behalf of the Union Internationale Centre de Cancer, Hayward et al (1977) defined criteria for objective assessment of response in advanced breast cancer, which have now been applied to the assessment of response in other tumour types. Reported methods of evaluating the response of bone metastases rely heavily on assessment of recalcification (healing) of previously lytic lesions. This does not directly measure shrinkage of the tumour mass or decrease in tumour activity, but merely the capacity for bone repair in areas previously destroyed by tumour cells. These traditional methods are those usually used to assess response in comparative trials, but they are poorly correlated with the clinical well-being of the patient, and would therefore appear to be of limited value for assessment of the results of palliative treatment of bone metastases (Nielsen et al, 1991). Newer methods for evaluating response in bone include biochemical markers of bone metabolism, tumour markers and measurements of symptomatic response (Coleman et al, 1988).

3.2 Breast Cancer

One-half of all breast cancer patients develop metastases at some time during the course of their disease and the skeleton is the most common site of distant recurrence. Bone metastases are identified clinically in approximately 70% of patients with advanced breast cancer and most of these metastases will require therapy (Costa et al, 1994). About 20% of patients with breast cancer have evidence of metastases only in bone (Nielsen et al, 1991). Once metastases have occurred, breast cancer is considered to be incurable and the goal of treatment for this metastatic disease is palliative. The median duration of survival for patients with metastatic breast cancer is brief: 2–3 years (Overmoyer,1995). Overall, patients with only bone metastases have the longest survival.

While the indications for local therapeutic modalities such as irradiation and surgery are well defined, much controversy persists concerning the use and the effects of systemic therapy of bone metastases. The application of chemotherapy for metastatic breast cancer has improved overall survival only modestly; nonetheless, the high response rate has effectively ameliorated many tumour-related symptoms. Chemotherapy has also increased treatment-related toxicity, often at the expense of quality of life (Overmoyer,1995). For this reason, patient selection is important in the decision to use chemotherapy as a method of palliation. Few specific criteria exist to guide the clinician in choosing chemotherapy over hormonal therapy as palliative treatment for metastatic breast cancer. In patients with rapidly progressive, symptomatic, life-threatening disease with visceral improvement and oestrogen-receptor-negative tumours, chemotherapy is the treatment of choice (Overmoyer, 1995). Hormonal therapy may be more appropriate for patients who have a more indolent form of the disease, or for asymptomatic patients who have a low tumour burden and positive hormonal receptors.

3.2.1 Response rates

Most phase II studies have investigated breast cancer patients with all manifestations of advanced disease. Thus, response of bone metastases to systemic therapy must be derived from the data presented and these generally refer to a limited number of patients. Moreover, objective response assessment in skeletal metastases is difficult. Reported response rates in bone are therefore highly variable and usually lower than in other sites. Among randomised studies the response rates in bone are generally low, varying between 0 and 41% (Costa et al, 1994; Perez et al, 1990). The bone pain in many patients responds promptly to chemotherapy (within 10–14 days), and pain relief may precede radiological changes by many months (Nielsen et al, 1991). Responses of bone metastases are nearly always partial, with a median duration of response of 9–16 months (Costa et al, 1994; Perez et al, 1990). The subgroup of patients with bone metastases only seems to have a favourable prognosis compared with patients with metastases in other sites, and their primary tumour is more commonly oestrogen-receptor-positive (Nielsen et al, 1991). Endocrine treatment has been reported to be effective in up to 85% of these patients. Combination chemotherapy has also been described as an effective treatment in this subgroup but is associated with a greater incidence of side-effects (Nielsen et al, 1991).

About two-thirds of all patients with metastatic breast cancer will have a response to some form of chemotherapy, although complete response rates in the range of 10–20% have been reported in most trials. The median duration of response to chemotherapy is 6–12 months (Nielsen et al, 1991).

3.2.2 Chemotherapeutic agents for breast cancer

The chemotherapeutic agents with the greatest efficacy against breast cancer are the alkylating agents and anthracyclines, producing response rates of 30–50% when administered as single agents (Hoogestraten and Fabian, 1979; Taylor and Gelber, 1982). Moreover, methotrexate and 5-fluorouracil demonstrated single-agent response rates of 26–28% (Carter, 1976.) Several studies have confirmed that combination chemotherapy is more effective in inducing responses compared with single-agent treatment, albeit at the cost of greater toxicity (Overmoyer, 1995). The most commonly used initial combination regimens include CMF (cyclophosphamide, methotrexate and fluorouracil), CAF or FAC (substituting doxorubicin for methotrexate in CMF), CEF (substituting epirubicin for methotrexate in CMF) and CNF (substituting mitoxantrone for methotrexate in CMF). Use of CMF in metastatic disease produces response rates of 46–66% (Overmoyer, 1995). The anthracycline-based regimen (FAC or FEC) reports response rates between 50 and 60% (Henderson, 1991). Doxorubicin-containing regimens induce higher response rates with prolonged median duration of response between 10 and 18 months, but the median survival time of 18–26 months is modestly superior to the most commonly used combination CMF (Sledge and Antman, 1992). When disease progresses despite initial therapy, vinca alkaloids (vincristine, vinblastine), mitomycin and other agents (etoposide, cisplatin, carboplatin, thiotepa) have been used.

These second-line chemotherapy agents generally produce a lower response rate with a short duration, measured in weeks to a few months. The emergence of new active agents such as vinorelbine (a semisynthetic non-vinca alkaloid agent) and the taxanes (paclitaxel and docetaxel) has provided a valuable alternative option for patients with metastatic breast cancer. Single-agent phase II trials of vinorelbine have yielded response rates of 40–60% in patients without prior therapy for stage IV disease and of 20–30% among patients with prior chemotherapy exposure (Seidman, 1996). Combination trials of vinorelbine with doxorubicin, epirubicin, mitoxantrone, paclitaxel, fluorouracil, mitomycin and other agents have reported response rates of 56–78% as first-line therapy and 18–45% as second- to third-line therapy. The most successful combinations included anthracyclines (Fumoleau et al, 1995).

3.2.2.1 *Paclitaxel*

Paclitaxel represents the first taxane. It promotes polymerisation of tubulin, increasing microtubule assembly and stabilising any microtubules already formed. This prevents the reorganisation of the microtubule network required to form the spindle during mitosis and therefore disrupts the distribution of chromosome into daughter cells, preventing cell replication. The single-agent response rate for paclitaxel in patients with minimal prior chemotherapy for advanced breast cancer is well above 50% (Hortobagyi and Holmes, 1996), with a stepwise decrement in activity noted in relation to the extent of prior chemotherapy received. Even in the "salvage" setting, in which extensive prior chemotherapy has been administered, a 23% response rate is noted (Hortobagyi and Holmes, 1996). Moreover, paclitaxel retains significant antitumour activity, even in anthracycline-resistant disease, with reported response rates of 26–42% (Nabholtz, 1996; Fountzilas, 1996). Most clinicians use a 3-hour schedule of administration and a dose of 175 mg/m^2. In second-line therapy, the active combination regimen of paclitaxel by 3-hour infusion with bolus doxorubicin is now commonly used (Gianni et al, 1995).

3.2.2.2 *Docetaxel*

Docetaxel is another effective anticancer agent of the same chemical class as paclitaxel. In phase II studies, docetaxel has shown significant anticancer activity as a first-line therapy for patients with metastatic breast cancer, achieving an overall response rate of 59% (Chevallier et al, 1995; van Oosterom, 1995). The role of docetaxel as monotherapy in patients with second-line metastatic breast cancer has been investigated in an extensive phase II clinical trial programme (Ravdin et al, 1995; Valero et al, 1995; ten Bokkel-Huinink et al, 1994). The overall response rate was 50% in non-anthracycline-resistant patients and 41% in anthracycline-resistant patients, and the median duration of response from the start of treatment was 6 months. These results compare favourably with current combination chemotherapy options for anthracycline-resistant metastatic breast cancer (van Oosterom, 1995). Preclinical data in mammary models have shown that a synergism between docetaxel and other chemotherapeutic agents may exist (Bissery et al, 1995). A growing number of clinical pilot studies are currently focusing on the combination of docetaxel and other drugs such as doxorubicin, fluorouracil, vinorelbine, cyclophosphamide or ifosfamide. Combinations of taxoids with vinca alkaloids appear promising and well tolerated, while the optimal way to combine these two classes of agents remains to be determined (Fumoleau et al, 1995; Piccart et al, 1996).

3.2.3 High-dose Chemotherapy and Haematocellular Support

For selected patients with metastatic disease that is responding to chemotherapeutic agents at conventional doses (clinically chemosensitive disease), the administration of high-dose chemotherapy with haematocellular support (e.g. autologous bone marrow transplantation or peripheral blood progenitor cell) represents an investigational approach that a growing number of physicians consider. Phase II data of high-dose chemotherapy with autologous haematopoietic progenitor cell support in metastatic breast cancer are promising, with results equivalent or superior to published reports using conventional chemotherapy (Bearman et al, 1996). Prospective randomised trials are ongoing to define the utility of high-dose chemotherapy in the treatment of chemosensitive stage IV breast disease.

The patient with metastatic breast cancer is best managed with the judicious use of local and systemic therapies that will achieve maximum palliation with minimal toxicity. Whenever systemic therapy is considered, an endocrine regimen should be used in patients with a more indolent course, oestrogen-receptor-positive tumours, a long disease-free interval, and soft-tissue or bone involvement. Chemotherapy is more appropriate as initial treatment in patients who do not have the above characteristics or those who have rapidly progressive disease, increasing symptoms or have failed to respond to endocrine therapy (Overmoyer, 1995).

3.3 Lung Cancer

3.3.1 Small-cell lung cancer (SCLC)

There are few other common solid tumours with osseous involvement in which chemotherapy is of proven value. In SCLC 50–80% of patients with bony symptoms may show pain relief after combination chemotherapy (Nielsen et al, 1991). Over the past two decades, a clear improvement in the median survival time of patients with extensive SCLC has occurred with the routine use of systemic chemotherapy. Today, such patients can expect a fourfold improvement in survival (Nielsen et al, 1991).

For much of the past two decades, CAV (cyclophosphamide, adriamycin, vincristine) has been the standard systemic therapy. This three-drug regimen has produced overall response rates ranging from 55 to 65%, including a 10–15% complete remission rate and a median survival of approximately 8 months (Loeher, 1995). In the 1980s, cisplatin plus etoposide (PE) emerged as a successful two-drug salvage regimen for patients with recurrent disease. Pooled data from several series reported overall response rates of approximately 50% in patients who had previously received CAV combination chemotherapy (Loeher, 1995). The median survival time of such patients was approximately 4 months. Numerous phase II trials have evaluated cisplatin plus etoposide as initial therapy and have confirmed the activity of this combination, achieving response rates and median survival times comparable to those reported for CAV (Loeher, 1995).

Recently, several new active drugs have been identified for treating patients with SCLC. These include paclitaxel, docetaxel, CPT-11, topotecan and gemcitabine. The response rates for paclitaxel, topotecan and gemcitabine given to previously untreated patients are 34–41%, 39% and 30% respectively. The response rates for docetaxel, CPT-11 and topotecan given to previously treated patients are 28%, 47% and 11–30% respectively (Johnson, 1995; Perez-Soler et al, 1996). Studies are needed to evaluate the efficacy of combination chemotherapy utilising these new agents either together or with other effective agents such as platinum analogue, etoposide and ifosfamide in the treatment of SCLC.

3.3.2 Non-small-cell Lung Cancer (NSCLC)

Up to 50% of patients with non-small cell-lung cancer (NSCLC) present with stage IV disease or metastatic disease, and 87% will ultimately die of their neoplasm (Adelstein, 1995). As such, chemotherapy will be considered for the majority at some point during their illness. Relatively few chemotherapeutic agents have demonstrated antitumour activity in NSCLC. The most active single agents (with response rates more than 20%) are cisplatin, ifosfamide and mitomycin (Adelstein, 1995). Cisplatin is generally considered to be the most important. This drug is a key ingredient of combination chemotherapy for stage IV.

In view of the finding that NSCLC is insensitive to chemotherapy, it has been questioned whether chemotherapy is justified in the treatment of metastatic NSCLC. Seven phase III studies have compared best supportive care with cisplatin-based chemotherapy. All seven trials demonstrated an improved median survival in patients receiving chemotherapy; however, this difference attained statistical significance in only three studies (Adelstein, 1995). A recently completed meta-analysis of these data has suggested that there is a small, short-lived survival benefit for patients given chemotherapy (Souquet et al, 1993). The median survival time for chemotherapy patients ranges from 20 to 34 weeks, compared with 9–21 weeks for patients who received best supportive care. However, the impact of chemotherapy on overall quality of life remains unclear.

For the first time, there are now a number of novel chemotherapeutic agents that show considerable promise in the treatment of NSCLC. The first is vinorelbine (Navelbine), a novel semisynthetic vinca alkaloid. Vinorelbine is the first drug approved by the Food and Drug Administration in over 20 years for the first-line treatment of ambulatory patients with unresectable advanced NSCLC. Across phase II trials, vinorelbine demonstrates remarkably consistent clinical effects in patients with NSCLC. The range in the objective response rate for vinorelbine as a single agent (from 12 to 33%) may reflect differences in patient populations or multicentre versus single-institution studies (Crawford, 1996). However, the impact on survival and 1-year survival has been remarkably consistent. In the US multicentre phase III trial, median survival for patients receiving vinorelbine was 30 weeks, with a 1-year survival rate of 25%, compared with 22 weeks for 5-fluorouracil and leucovorin, with a 1-year survival rate of 16% (Crawford et al, 1996). This impact on survival was confirmed in a large European multicentre randomised trial. In this study, vinorelbine as a single agent demonstrated a median survival of 31 weeks, with a 1-year survival rate of 30% (Chevallier et al, 1994). Furthermore, in the largest randomised phase III trial, the addition of cisplatin to vinorelbine significantly improved these survival results (median survival rate of 40 weeks, 1-year survival rate of 35%).

Other new promising agents in NSCLC are paclitaxel, docetaxel, CPT-11 and gemcitabine. Phase II trials of single-agent paclitaxel in NSCLC have reported response rates of 21–24%. Docetaxel is most commonly administered at doses of 80–100 mg/m^2 by a 1-h infusion, repeated every 3 weeks. Results of phase II trials in NSCLC have shown response rates of 25–38% to single-agent docetaxel with prolonged duration of responses (Edelman and Gandara, 1996). Significant clinical activity of CPT-11 has been demonstrated in phase II trials in NSCLC (Fukuoka et al, 1992). Subsequent Japanese trials have combined CPT-11 with cisplatin or cisplatin/vindesine, with response rates ranging from 40 to 54% (Edelman and Gandara, 1996). Preliminary results from several phase II trials with gemcitabine in advanced NSCLC have reported response rates of 20–30% (Edelman et al, 1996). Despite encouraging results, the exact role that these new agents will play in the therapy of NSCLC remains unclear.

3.4 Prostate Cancer

The natural history of hormone-resistant prostatic cancer has remained unaltered, with a median survival of only approximately 12 months. In prostate cancer, the assessment of response is particularly difficult and many groups (National Prostatic Cancer Project, World Health Organization, European Organization for Research and Treatment of Cancer) have tried to use a combination of changes in radiography, bone scintigraphy, acid phosphatase, performance status and symptoms (Aabo, 1987). These methods suffer from being subjective, and evaluation of response by bone scintigraphy is difficult (Aabo, 1987). Recently, a decline in prostate-specific antigen (PSA) has been advocated as an intermediate marker of response, and as a surrogate marker for survival in patients with hormone-refractory prostate cancer, although controversy remains (Eisenberger and Nelson, 1996).

A number of promising new approaches have been tested recently and brought to trial, including combined antimicrotubular therapy (estramustine-based therapy), camptothecins, suramin, mitoxantrone and doxorubicin-based regimens. These new non-hormonal agents have demonstrated activity and remain as options in the treatment of patients with truly hormone-refractory prostate cancer.

3.4.1 Estramustine

The synthetic agent estramustine phosphate has been widely used in the treatment of advanced prostatic carcinoma. It has demonstrated a modest single-agent activity with an overall response rate of 4.6% (Murphy et al, 1983). Randomised trials comparing single-agent estramustine to other therapies failed to show any obvious benefit (Roth, 1996).

An understanding of the mechanism of action of estramustine, which binds to microtubule-associated proteins, has prompted trials combining estramustine with other antimicrotubular agents, including vinblastine, vinorelbine and, more recently, paclitaxel. The three phase II studies of the combination of estramustine plus vinblastine have suggested some degree of activity, with approximately 46–61% of patients showing at least a 50% reduction in PSA and 16–32% of patients showing at least an 80% reduction in PSA, and some partial responses in patients with measurable disease (Roth, 1996). Despite the remarkable similarity of these phase II results and the suggestion of synergy, phase III trials are in progress to define the role of combined estramustine plus vinblastine anti-microtubular therapy.

The phase II trial of the Eastern Cooperative Oncology Group with single-agent paclitaxel, either at 170 mg/m^2 or 135 mg/m^2, as a 24-h continuous infusion, for patients with extensive prior radiotherapy showed only modest single-agent activity for paclitaxel. In this study, 4.3% of patients experienced a partial response rate of nodal disease associated with an 80% reduction in serum PSA for a period of 9 months (Roth et al, 1993). Based on these findings, Hudes et al. conducted a phase II study of the combination of estramustine and paclitaxel given as a 96-h continuous infusion, which demonstrated activity (Hudes et al, 1995a). In 16 patients with bone- only disease, 11 (68.8%) had at least a 50% reduction in serum PSA and six (37.5%) had at least an 80% reduction in PSA from baseline. Moreover, for the 24 evaluable patients, the PSA response proportion (65%) and objective response proportion (50%) are encouraging, but small numbers of patients and the confounding use of high-dose steroids required as premedication for paclitaxel, indicate the need for additional study of this regimen.

The only published phase II trial in advanced prostate cancer utilising a topoisomerase I inhibitor used topotecan and involved 34 evaluable patients. In this study topotecan showed some modest single-agent activity (Hudes et al, 1995b).

3.4.2 Suramin

Suramin is the first of a new class of growth factor antagonists. The efficacy of suramin has not been established, because of different schedules and doses used and because of vastly different study entry criteria. Approximately 50% of patients treated with suramin achieve a PSA response, with some long-term survivors reported (Reyno et al, 1995), although some investigators are less optimistic about this new agent (Kelly et al, 1995). Nevertheless, major toxicities of suramin include neurotoxicity, myelosuppression, fatigue, anorexia, fever and peripheral oedema. Moreover, suramin frequently causes adrenocortical insufficiency, therefore hydrocortisone replacement therapy is commonly used. The confounding role of steroids in assessing the efficacy of suramin is currently being evaluated by an intergroup randomised phase III study comparing suramin plus hydrocortisone to placebo plus hydrocortisone.

3.4.3 Mitoxantrone

Two groups of investigators have evaluated the efficacy of corticosteroids alone compared with corticosteroids plus mitoxantrone. The randomised study of mitoxantrone plus prednisone versus prednisone alone, initiated by Tannock et al (1996), is the first study to document an advantage to chemotherapy in hormone-refractory prostate cancer. The advantages observed were in pain control and duration of palliation, and not in survival. The authors reported a significant reduction in pain in 29% of patients treated with mitoxantrone plus prednisone compared with 12% of those treated with prednisone alone ($p<0.01$); the duration of palliation was longer in the mitoxantrone group (43 weeks versus 18 weeks, $p<0.0001$). The median survival (about 11 months) was the same in both treatment groups. It is clear that the use of mitoxantrone was palliative (Small et al, 1996).

3.4.4 Doxorubicin

Doxorubicin-based regimens have been used extensively in hormone-refractory prostate cancers. Phase II trials have reported an overall response rate of approximately 10%. More recently, the use of doxorubicin in combination with dose-escalated cyclophosphamide has been reported, with an objective response proportion of 33% and a PSA response proportion of approximately 50%. Some dramatic bone scan responses, computed tomography responses and long-term PSA responses were observed; toxicity seemed reasonable (Small et al, 1996).

Thus, a host of new agents with demonstrable activity against prostate cancer are being developed and brought to clinical study. Nevertheless, the prostate cancer patient population tends to be old, with low performance status and their tolerance of toxic chemotherapeutic regimens is often poor. Ideally, patients should receive chemotherapy only within a clinical trial. So, when a patient with a good performance status has symptomatic progressive metastatic disease after appropriate initial therapy, followed by anti-androgen withdrawal and an appropriate secondary hormonal manipulation, it is appropriate to consider active chemotherapeutic agents and experimental agents in a well-designed phase I or phase II clinical trial.

3.5 Renal Cell Carcinoma

Approximately 25% of patients with renal cell carcinoma develop bony metastases (Coleman, 1994). The treatment of patients with renal cell carcinoma continues to be disappointing. A number of promising new approaches have been tested recently, with poor and non-reproducible results. The most extensively studied are vinblastine and floxuridine. The conventional chemotherapeutic treatment of metastatic renal cell carcinoma is vinblastine, 0.1–0.3 mg/kg per week. In a review of results achieved with this drug in 626 patients enrolled into 15 phase II studies, a median response rate of 17.5% was reported (Canobbio et al, 1996). Efforts to improve the response rate to vinblastine by administering it by continuous infusion have been largely unsuccessful (Canobbio et al, 1996). The clinical experience obtained with vincristine or semisynthetic analogues of vinblastine, such as vindesine and vinorelbine, is more limited. However, these drugs have not shown any relevant therapeutic activity (Canobbio et al, 1996). Floxuridine may have minimal but consistent antitumour activity ranging between 9 and 20%, but the responses are generally partial and relatively brief (Miglietta et al, 1994; Bjarson et al, 1994).

Newer agents such as carboplatin, ifosfamide, amsacrine, paclitaxel, fotemustine and suramin have all undergone phase II studies as potential agents against metastatic renal cell carcinoma, but to date they have shown no activity greater than vinblastine (Yagoda et al, 1995). Moreover, the use of combination chemotherapy has not yielded better results than the use of single agents, despite an increase in toxicity (Motzer et al, 1995). Agents that reverse the multidrug resistance associated with P-glycoprotein, including verapamil and cylosporin, have not enhanced the antitumour effect of vinblastine (Motzer et al, 1995). Therefore, the study of new agents is indicated in patients who have never had chemotherapy. Systemic therapy for metastatic renal cell carcinoma should be administered, whenever possible, in the context of a clinical trial. At the moment immunotherapy remains the most effective approach to the treatment of metastatic renal cell carcinoma.

3.6 Summary

Bone metastases are frequently one of the first signs of disseminated disease in cancer patients and a major source of morbidity. In the majority of patients, the primary tumour is in the breast, prostate or lung. The optimum systemic treatment for bone metastases depends on the tumour type. This chapter concentrated on chemotherapy of breast, lung, prostate and renal cancer. Chemotherapy is demonstrably effective in the treatment of bone metastases in malignancies such as breast cancer and SCLC. In metastatic breast cancer, chemotherapy is reserved for endocrine-resistant or rapidly progressive life-threatening visceral disease. The application of chemotherapy for this metastatic cancer has modestly improved overall survival; nonetheless, the high response rate has effectively ameliorated many tumour-related symptoms.

Over the past two decades, a clear improvement in the median survival time of patients with extensive SCLC has occurred with the routine use of systemic chemotherapy. Today, such patients can expect a fourfold improvement in survival. In NSCLC, the results with chemotherapy have been poor. There are now promising new chemotherapeutic agents in the treatment of NSCLC, such as taxanes, vinorelbine, CPT-11, topotecan and gemcitabine.

In the treatment of patients with truly hormone-refractory prostate cancer, promising new approaches have been tested recently. These new non-hormonal agents have demonstrated activity and remain as options in the treatment of these patients. The treatment of patients with renal cell carcinoma continues to be disappointing. A number of promising new approaches have been tested recently, with poor and non-reproducible results.

References

Aabo K (1987) Prostate cancer: evaluation of response to treatment, response criteria, and need for standardization of the reporting of results. Eur J Cancer Clin Oncol 23:231–236.

Adelstein DJ (1995) Palliative chemotherapy for non-small cell lung cancer. Semin Oncol 22(suppl 3):35–39.

Bearman SI, Shpall EJ, Jones RB et al (1996) High-dose chemotherapy with autologous hematopoietic progenitor cell support for metastatic and high-risk primary breast cancer. Semin Oncol 23(suppl 2):60–67.

Bissery MC, Nohynek G, Sanderink GJ (1995) Docetaxel (taxotere Rm): a review of preclinical experience. Part 1: preclinical experience. Anticancer Drugs 6:339–368.

Bjarson G, Hrushesky WJ, Diasio R et al. (1994) Flat versus circadian modified 14 day infusion of FUDR for advanced renal cell cancer (RCC): a phase-III study. Proc Am Soc Clin Oncol 1:718 (Abstract 233).

Canobbio L, Miglietta L, Boccardo F (1996) Medical treatment of advanced renal cell carcinoma: present option and future directions. Cancer Treatment Review 22:85–104.

Carter SK (1976) Integration of chemotherapy into combined modality treatment of solid tumours. Cancer Treatment Review 3:141–174.
Chevallier B, Pujol JL, Douillard JY et al (1994) Randomized study of vinorelbine and cisplatin vs vindesine and cisplatin vs vinorelbine alone in advanced non-small cell lung cancer: results of a European multicenter trial including 612 patients. J Clin Oncol 12:360–367.
Chevallier B, Fumoleau P, Kerbrat P et al (1995) Docetaxel is a major cytotoxic drug for the treatment of advanced breast cancer: a phase II trial of the Clinical Screening Cooperative Group of the European Organization for Research and Treatment of Cancer. J Clin Oncol 13:314–322.
Coleman RE, Whitaker KD, Moss DW et al (1998) Biochemical monitoring predicts response in bone metastases to treatment. Br J Cancer 55:61–66.
Coleman R (1994) Incidence and distribution of bone metastases. In: Diel IJ, Kaufmann M, Bastert G (eds) Metastatic bone disease. Springer-Verlag, Heidelberg, pp 20–30.
Costa SD, Diel IJ, Solomayer E (1994) Systemic treatment of bone metastasis: review of the literature and retrospective analysis of 718 breast cancer patients. In: Diel IJ, Kaufmann M, Bastert G (eds) Metastatic bone disease. Springer-Verlag, Heidelberg, pp 133–143.
Crawford J (1996) Update: vinorelbine (Navelbine) in non-small cell lung cancer. Semin Oncol 23(suppl 5):2–7.
Crawford J, O'Rourke M, Schiller JH et al. (1996) Randomized trial of vinorelbine compared with fluorouracil plus leucovorin in patients with stage IV non-small-cell lung cancer. J Clin Oncol 14:2774–2784.
Edelman MJ, Gandara DR (1996) Promising new agents in the treatment of non-small cell lung cancer. Cancer Chemother Pharmacol 37:385–393.
Eisenberger MA, Nelson WG (1996) How much can we rely on the level of prostate-specific antigen as an end point for evaluation of clinical trials? A word of caution! J Natl Cancer Inst 88:779–781.
Fountzilas G (1996) A phase II study of paclitaxel in advanced breast cancer resistant to anthracyclines. Eur J Cancer 32A:47–51.
Fukuoka M, Niitani H, Suzuki A et al (1992) A phase II study of CPT-11, a new derivative camptothecin for previously untreated non-small-cell lung cancer. J Clin Oncol 10:16.
Fumoleau P, Delozier JM, Extra L et al (1995) Vinorelbine (Navelbine) in the treatment of breast cancer: the European experience. Semin Oncol 22(suppl. 5):22–29.
Gianni L, Munzone E, Capri G et al (1995) Paclitaxel by 3-hour infusion in combination with bolus doxorubicin in women with untreated metastatic breast cancer: high antitumour efficacy and cardiac effects in a dose-finding and sequence-finding study. J Clin Oncol 13:2688–2699.
Hayward JL, Carbone PP, Heuson JC et al (1977) Assessment of response to therapy in advanced breast cancer. Eur J Cancer 13:89–94.
Henderson IC (1991) Chemotherapy for metastatic disease. In: Harris S, Hellman S, Henderson IC, Kinne D, (eds) Breast disease, 2nd edn. JB Lippincott, Philadelphia, pp 604–665.
Hoogestraten B, Fabian C (1979) A reappraisal of single drugs to advanced breast cancer. Cancer Clinical Trials 2:101–198.
Hortobagyi GN, Holmes FA (1996) Single-agent paclitaxel for the treatment of breast cancer: an overview. Semin Oncol 23(suppl 1):4–9.
Hudes GR, Nathan FE, Khater C et al. (1995a) Paclitaxel plus estramustine in metastatic hormone-refractory prostate cancer. Semin Oncol 22:41–45.
Hudes GR, Kosierowski R, Greenberg R et al. (1995b) Phase II study of topotecan in metastatic hormone refractory-prostate cancer. Investigational New Drugs 13:235–240.
Johnson DH. (1995) Future directions in the management of small-cell lung cancer. Lung Cancer 12(suppl. 3):S71–75.
Kelly W, Curley T, Leibertz G et al (1995) Prospective evaluation of hydrocortisone and suramin in patients with androgen-independent prostate cancer. J Clin Oncol 13:2208–2213.
Loeher PJ (1995) Palliative therapy: extensive small cell lung cancer. Semin Oncol 22(suppl 3):40–44.
Marty M. (1994) Place des traitements spécifiques dans le traitement des douleurs associées au cancer. In: Serrie A, Thurel C (eds) La douleur en pratique quotidienne. Arnette, Paris, pp 447–469.
Miglietta L, Canobbio L, Cannata D et al (1994) Low activity of circadian continuous fluorodeoxyuridine (FUDR) chemotherapy in poor prognosis metastatic renal cancer. Oncology Report 1:121–123.
Motzer RJ, Lyn P, Fisher P et al (1995) Phase I/II trial of dexverapamil plus vinblastine for patients with advanced renal cell carcinoma. J Clin Oncol 13:1958–1965.
Murphy JP, Slack NH, Mittelman A (1983) Experiences with estramustine phosphate in prostate cancer. Semin Oncol 12:689–694.
Nabholtz JM (1996) Multicenter randomized comparative study of two doses of paclitaxel in patients with metastatic breast cancer. J Clin Oncol 14:1858–1867
Nielsen OS, Alastair JM, Tannock IF (1991) Bone metastases: pathophysiology and management policy. J Clin Oncol 9:509–524.

Overmoyer BA (1995) Chemotherapeutic palliative approaches in the treatment of breast cancer. Semin Oncol 22(suppl 3):2–9.

Perez JE, Machiavelli M, Leone BA et al (1990) Bone-only versus visceral-only metastatic pattern in breast cancer: analysis of 150 patients. Am J Clin Oncol 13(4):294–298.

Perez-Soler R, Glisson BS, Lee JS et al. (1996) Treatment of patients with small-cell lung cancer refractory to etoposide and cisplatin with the topoisomerase I poison topotecan. J Clin Oncol 14:2785–2790.

Piccart M, Di Leo A, De Variola A et al (1996) Docetaxel in the treatment of breast cancer: current status, ongoing trials and future directions. In: Calvo F, Crépin M, Magdelenat H (eds) Breast cancer advances in biology and therapeutics. John Libbey Eurotext, Montrouge, pp 257–264.

Ravdin PM, Burris HA, Cook G et al (1995) Phase II trial of docetaxel in advanced anthracyclin-resistant or anthracenedione-resistant breast cancer. J Clin Oncol 13:2879–2885.

Reyno LE, Egorin MJ, Eisenberger MA et al (1995) Development and validation of a pharmacokinetically based fixed dosing scheme for suramin. J Clin Oncol 13:2187–2195.

Roth BJ, Yeap BY, Wilding GW et al (1993) Taxol in advanced hormone-refractory carcinoma of the prostate. Cancer 72:2457–2460.

Roth BJ (1996) New therapeutic agents for hormone-refractory prostate cancer. Semin Oncol 23(suppl 14):49–55.

Seidman A (1996) Chemotherapy for advanced breast cancer: a current perspective. Semin Oncol 23(suppl 2):55–59.

Sledge GW, Antman KH (1992) Progress in chemotherapy for metastatic breast cancer. Semin Oncol 19:317–332.

Small ES, Scrinivas S, Egan B et al. (1996) Doxorubicin and dose-escalated cyclophosphamide with granulocyte colony-stimulating factor for the treatment of hormone-resistant prostate cancer. J Clin Oncol 14:1617–1625.

Souquet PJ, Chauvin F, Boissel JP et al (1993) Polychemotherapy in advanced non-small cell lung cancer. A meta-analysis. Lancet 342:19–21.

Tannock I, Osoba D, Stocker MR et al (1996) Chemotherapy with mitoxantrone plus prednisone or prenisone alone for symptomatic hormone resistant prostate cancer: a Canadian randomized trial with palliative end points. J Clin Oncol 14:11756–11764.

Taylor SGIV, Gelber R (1982) Experience of the Eastern Cooperative Oncology Working Group with doxorubicin as a single agent in patients with previously untreated breast cancer. Cancer Treatment Report 66:1594–1595.

ten Bokkel-Huinink WW, Prove AM, Piccart M et al (1994) A phase II trial with docetaxel (Taxotere) in second line treatment with chemotherapy for advanced breast cancer. A study of the EORTC Early Clinical Screening group. Ann Oncol 5:527–532.

Valero V, Holmes FA, Walters RS et al (1995) Phase II trial of docetaxel: a new, highly effective antineoplastic agent in the management of patients with anthracyclin-resistant metastatic breast cancer. J Clin Oncol 13:2886–2894.

Van Oosterom AT (1995) Docetaxel (Taxotere): an effective agent in the management of second line breast cancer. Semin Oncol 22(suppl 13):22–28.

Yagoda A, Abi-Rached B, Petrylak D (1995) Chemotherapy for advanced renal-cell carcinoma: 1983–1993. Semin Oncol 22:42–60.

4 Immunotherapy

Th. Dorval

Foley (1953) was the first to demonstrate that the immune system is capable of rejecting tumours. He showed that immunisation of mice against tumour cells prevented the uptake of lethal doses of tumour cells. This experiment opened the way for studies on immunotherapy for cancer in humans.

The rapid increase in immunological knowledge and the development of techniques in molecular biology have stimulated studies on the possibility and efficacy of immunotherapy for cancer. Such a therapeutic approach can be divided into active and passive immunotherapy.

Active immunotherapy refers to the immunisation of the patient with materials supposed to induce an immune reaction capable of eliminating or retarding tumour growth. Active immunotherapy can be divided into non-specific and specific immunotherapy. Non-specific active approaches have been used for decades in the treatment of cancer with adjuvants such as bacillus Calmette-Guérin (BCG) injections, *Corynebacterium parvum* extracts and levamisole. Specific active immunotherapy uses immunisation with tumour cell extracts alone or vaccines, often in conjunction with modulators such as BCG. These early approaches have never demonstrated any benefit and have largely been abandoned.

The recent description of tumour antigens expressed by tumour cells led to the development of new strategies aimed at stimulating antitumour immunity. Recently, the advent of recombinant techniques has allowed production of large amounts of cytokines and has rekindled interest in the biological therapy of tumours. Treatment with interferon or interleukin-2 is a form of non-specific active immunotherapy and the selective action of these lymphokines allows a greater ability to manipulate immune response than was previously possible. Until the tumour-bearing host is immunosuppressed, active immunotherapy may have intrinsic disadvantages.

Passive approaches to immunotherapy have been developed, which involve the transfer of previously sensitised immunological agents that have the ability to mediate immune antitumour response. Recent efforts have been devoted to developing immunotherapy using ex-vivo stimulated cells (lymphokine-activated killer cells, tumour-infiltrating lymphocytes). Concurrently, the development of new techniques to generate monoclonal antibodies has improved the ability to obtain preparations with specific reactivity to tumour-associated antigens. Clinical experience of immunotherapy in cancer patients is very limited; it has proven to be of benefit only in the treatment of renal cell cancer and malignant melanoma. In those tumours, objective responses have been reported, including responses in patients with bone metastases.

The place of immunotherapy in the treatment of bone metastases is very limited, as immunotherapy is applied only in renal cell cancer and metastatic melanoma. Moreover, immunotherapy is never the sole treatment of bone metastases. It is usually given for diffuse metastatic disease.

4.1 Active Non-specific Immunotherapy

The rationale for early attempts to perform immunotherapy was to stimulate the immune system non-specifically, with the hope that a non-specific increase in immune reactivity would lead to a concomitant increase in immune reaction to established tumours (Hersh and Taylor, 1991).

Bacterial toxins have been administered and anecdotal observations have been reported by Coley and other authors. These encouraging results have not been repeated successfully, but have led to extensive studies of the use of non-specific immunotherapy in experimental and human cancer. A wide variety of "immunomodulating" agents have been tested, including bacteria, bacterial products and purified compounds.

In animal models, BCG improves immune reaction, with increased antibody formation and accelerated graft rejection, and has been used in many early studies. Human cancers have been treated with BCG given as an adjuvant and in patients with metastatic disease. These first non-randomised studies suggested some efficacy of immunotherapy and led to prospective randomised trials.

Active non-specific immunotherapy has been unsuccessful in the treatment of patients with advanced disease; the initial encouraging results have not been confirmed in prospective randomised trials and these approaches have been abandoned.

Some trials have tested BCG therapy as an adjuvant. Historical positive results could not be confirmed in prospective randomised trials. This therapy has demonstrated some efficacy when administered locally in metastatic melanoma and in bladder cancer. This technique cannot be applied to bone metastases.

4.2 Active Specific Immunotherapy

Successful prevention of bacterial and viral diseases by immunisation led to the hope that immunisation against tumour cells could induce the regression of established tumours. Attempts to develop tumour vaccines included immunisation with autologous or allogeneic tumour cells alone or in combination with immune adjuvants such as BCG. No models of active specific immunotherapy have been effective in animals; nevertheless, the absence of animal models did not stop clinical trials in the treatment of human tumours being undertaken. This therapeutic approach has been tested in a variety of tumours, including leukaemia, melanoma, osteosarcoma, renal cell cancer, ovarian cancer, using a variety of immunisation schedules (Hoover and Hanna, 1991). Although objective regressions have been reported, the reproducibility of these results remains uncertain and this approach has been abandoned in advanced disease. Some trials are still ongoing in the prevention of relapse.

The recent discovery of the molecular structure of tumour antigens may contribute to the development of more specific and more efficient strategies (Traversari et al, 1992).

4.3 Passive Immunotherapy

Passive immunotherapy is represented by the use of monoclonal antibodies. These are characterised by a relatively unique antitumour specificity and there have been many attempts to use them in cancer treatment. Antibodies can be used alone or combined with various agents, such as drugs, toxins or radionuclides. The advantages of this approach are the relative specificity of the antibodies for the tumour and the absence of toxicity associated with their administration. The clinical experience is limited and no conclusion can yet be drawn (Drebin et al, 1995). The major problem with the use of murine monoclonal antibodies is the development of human antimouse antibodies, which inactivate the injected antibodies. New techniques have been developed and could circumvent this problem.

4.4 Interferons

The interferons are a family of proteins produced by cells in response to viral infection or stimulation with antigens, mitogens or double-stranded RNA. The interferons have antiviral properties but also have immunomodulatory and antiproliferative effects. There are three major groups of interferons: α, β and γ.

Interferon? α can be produced by a variety of cells, including macrophages and lymphocytes, interferon β is produced by fibroblasts and epithelial cells, and interferon γ is produced by a variety of lymphocyte subtypes. Interferons have several biological properties, including immunomodulatory activities, antiviral activities, regulation of differentiation, inhibition of angiogenesis, and the ability to interfere with cell proliferation and to modulate the expression of cell-surface antigens. The antitumour activity of interferon results from its direct antiproliferative effect, but other properties may also be important.

The interferons have antitumour activity against a variety of tumours, including haematological and solid tumours (Borden, 1984). In solid tumours, interferon has demonstrated a modest but definite and reproducible activity in renal cell cancer and in metastatic melanoma. In most clinical trials, patients received recombinant 2 interferon.

In renal cell cancer, the objective response rate is about 10%, ranging from 5 to 25% (Muss, 1991). Sites of response include bone, but metastatic sites such as lung, lymph nodes or skin are more likely to respond to treatment. Response duration is usually short. Moreover, the effects of interferons on bone are usually difficult to evaluate, as most patients receive radiotherapy. The usual dose of interferon is 18 μ/m^2 subcutaneously, three times a week.

In metastatic melanoma, the objective response rate is 16% (Legha, 1989). Non-visceral, slowly growing tumour sites are more likely to respond to therapy but bone responses have been reported. Response is usually short, but long-lasting effects have been described. The given dose is 9–10 μ/m^2 subcutaneously, three times a week.

Toxicity is consistent but usually tolerable and does necessitate stopping therapy in most patients. It is represented by an influenza-like syndrome with fever, chills, arthralgia and myalgia. These symptoms start within 2 or 3 hours after injection, last for 6–12 hours and can be partially prevented by the administration of acetaminophen. All general side-effects usually abate slowly and disappear within the first month of treatment. Biological toxicity may be observed during the first 2 or 3 weeks of therapy and consists of an increase in liver enzymes and a decrease in blood count.

Interferon has been tested in combination with chemotherapeutic agents. However, initial encouraging results have not been not confirmed by prospective randomised trials (Falkson et al, 1991).

4.5 Interleukin-2

Interleukin-2 (IL-2) is a lymphokine produced by activated T cells. It has pleiotropic actions and plays a central role in immune regulation. It is capable of stimulating the growth of activated T cells that bear the IL-2 receptor; it also has other actions on T cells, B cells, macrophages and other cells. Large amounts of IL-2 can be produced, as the gene coding for human IL-2 has been coded and expressed in bacteria.

Interleukin-2 alone exhibits antitumour activity in many animal models. This activity is dose- and schedule-dependent and is impaired in animals with a defective immune system, whatever the cause. Unlike interferon, IL-2 has no direct activity on cancer cells.

The greatest efficacy has been noted with schedules yielding sustained lower levels of IL-2, rather than brief high peak levels. Continuous infusion of IL-2 is considerably more active in a murine model of IL-2 therapy. The efficacy of IL-2 therapy in immune-competent animals is dependent on the immunogenicity of the tumour and the tumour burden.

Interleukin-2 has been tested in many human tumours and has demonstrated some efficacy in renal cell cancer and in metastatic melanoma.

Initial experience by Rosenberg and colleagues (1987) used very high doses of IL-2 and lymphokine-activated killer (LAK) cells. Lymphokine-activated killer cells are generated by incubating human peripheral blood lymphocytes with IL-2 for 3–4 days and are capable of lysing fresh tumour cells. The nature of the determinants recognised on fresh tumour by LAK cells is unknown but fresh normal cells do not appear to bear cell-surface determinants recognised by LAK cells.

Clinical trials using IL-2 and LAK cells were developed, as no antitumour responses were seen in early trials using LAK cells alone. Patients underwent daily leukapheresis for 3–5 consecutive days. The cells were cultured in vitro for 3–4 days with IL-2 and reinfused. Bolus injections of IL-2 were given every 8 hours at a dose of 100,000 units/kg body weight for 5 days, starting on the day of the first infusion of LAK cells. Two to four cycles were administered. In the first trial, 11 out of 25 patients with renal cell cancer or metastatic melanoma had objective tumour regression. Complete response was observed in one patient with metastatic melanoma. These initial encouraging results were promising, as all patients had advanced metastatic disease resistant to conventional therapies. Further trials have been activated in patients presenting with renal cell cancer or metastatic melanoma. The results of these trials did not confirm the initial results and were somewhat disappointing, with objective response rates in renal cancer or melanoma ranging from 3 to 56%. Approximately 15–20% of patients with these tumours obtain partial remission and about 5% complete remission, including durable responses. Responses have been reported in all tumour locations, including bone metastases.

Treatment schedules have been modified and the infusion of LAK cells has been abandoned, as the administration of IL-2 alone has the same efficacy. Other authors have administered IL-2 as a continuous infusion to decrease toxicity (West et al, 1987).

The administration of high-dose IL-2 is associated with substantial dose-limiting toxicity. The mechanism of toxicity is probably attributable to lymphoid infiltrates in vital organs. A vascular permeability leak leads to fluid retention and interstitial oedema, which in turn may lead to respiratory distress, weight gain and renal dysfunction. The side-effects of IL-2 are completely reversible after administration ceases. Nevertheless, the toxicity caused by high doses of IL-2 is a major problem.

Typically, IL-2 administration is associated with a drop in systemic vascular resistance, leading to tachycardia, decreased arterial blood pressure and an increase in cardiac index. The capillary leak results in weight gain, decreased diuresis and raised serum creatinine level, probably because of prerenal azotemia. Vasopressors are often used to prevent and limit the need for fluid replacement, which contributes to the interstitial oedema. The treatment-related mortality ranges from 1 to 3%.

In an attempt to decrease toxicity, low doses of IL-2 have been administered subcutaneously in patients with metastatic melanoma and appear to have the same efficacy as high doses of IL-2 in patients with renal cell cancer. No definite conclusion can be drawn, as no randomised trial has yet been conducted (Richards et al, 1992).

In an attempt to increase efficacy, IL-2 has been combined with interferon and/or cytotoxic agents. Some authors have reported higher response rates without any definite benefit in response duration or median survival.

4.6 Conclusion

The role of immunotherapy in the treatment of cancer is very limited and restricted to the use of interferon and IL-2. Objective responses in bone metastases have been observed in renal cell cancer and metastatic melanoma. The objective response rate has not been defined, as responses have not been analysed by site of response. New approaches using more specific agents would lead to better results.

References

Borden EC (1984) Progress towards therapeutic application of interferons. Cancer 54:2770–2776.

Coley WB (1982) The treatment of malignant tumors by repeated inoculations of erysipelas, with a report of original cases. Am J Med Sci 105:487–511.

Drebin JA, Link VC, Stern DF et al (1995) Down regulation of an oncogene protein product and reversion of the transformed phenotype by monoclonal antibodies. Cell 41:695–706.

Falkson C, Falkson G, Falkson H (1991) Improved results with the addition of interferon alfa-2a to dacarbazine in the treatment of patients with metastatic malignant melanoma. J Clin Oncol 9:1403–1408.

Foley EJ (1953) Antigenic properties of methylcholenthrene-induced tumours in mice of the strain of origin. Cancer Res 13:835–883.

Hersh EM, Taylor CW (1991) Immunotherapy by active immunization. In: De Vita VT, Hellman S, Rosenberg SA (eds) Biological therapy of cancer. JB Lippincott, Philadelphia, pp 613–626.

Hoover HC Jr, Hanna MG Jr (1991) Immunotherapy by active immunization. In: De Vita VT, Hellman S, Rosenberg SA (eds) Biological therapy of cancer. JB Lippincott, Philadelphia, pp 670–681.

Legha S (1989) Current therapy for malignant melanoma. Semin Oncol 16:34–44.

Muss HB (1991) The use of interferon in renal cell carcinoma. Eur J Cancer 27(suppl 4):84–87.

Richards JM, Mehta M, Ramming K et al (1992) Sequential chemoimmunotherapy in the treatment of metastatic melanoma. J Clin Oncol 10:1338–1343.

Rosenberg SA, Lotze MT, Muul ML et al (1987) A progress report on the treatment of 157 patients with advanced cancer using lymphokine-activated killer cells and interleukin-2 or high dose interleukin-2 alone. N Engl J Med 15:889–897.

Traversari C, Van Der Bruggen P, Luesher IF et al (1992) A nonapeptide encoded by human gene MAGE-1 is recognized on HLA-A1 by cytolytic T lymphocytes directed against tumour antigene MZ2-E. J Exp Med 176(5):1453–1457.

West WH, Tauer KW, Yannelli JR et al (1987) Constant infusion recombinant interleukin-2 in adoptive immunotherapy of advanced cancer. N Engl J Med 15:898–906.

5 Biphosphonates

F. Duffaud and R. Favre

5.1 Mechanism of Action

The biphosphonates have a phosphate–carbon–phosphate backbone, which binds tightly to calcified bone matrix. This core structure allows many possible variations by changing side chains or by esterifiyng phosphate groups. Many biphosphonates have been synthesised, with different chemical and biological characteristics.

Clodronate acts directly on mature osteoclasts and can have cytotoxic effects at the concentration necessary to suppress bone resorption. However, nitrogen-containing biphosphonates such as pamidronate are not toxic to osteoclasts at therapeutic concentrations (Reitsma et al, 1982). For pamidronate, the principal site of action is believed to reside in the terminal differentiation and final activation of osteoclasts (Löwik et al, 1988).

Biphosphonates inhibit osteoclast-mediated bone resorption; their potency depends on their structure. The exact mechanisms of inhibition of bone resorption are still not clear. Recent findings suggest that osteoblasts, at least those lining the bone surface, could be the essential target cells for biphosphonates, with secondary effects on the osteoclasts, probably by a change in the secretion of osteoclast-controlling factors (Sahni et al, 1993; Body et al, 1996). The relative importance of this osteoblast-dependent inhibitory activity of biphosphonates compared to a direct inhibition of osteoclast activity or secretory capacity remains to be determined (Body et al, 1996).

Biphosphonates can also induce osteoclast apoptosis (programmed cell death), as evaluated by cytoplasmic contraction, chromatin condensation and nuclear fragmentation, both in vitro and in vivo. This effect could also be mediated through the osteoblasts; for example, through stimulation of tissue growth factor secretion, which induces osteoclast apoptosis (Hughes et al, 1995). Many mechanisms are likely to be operating, varing from one individual compound to another.

The introduction of biphosphonates has dramatically changed the therapeutic management of tumour-induced hypercalcemia (Body, 1992; Ralston, 1992). These agents are now the standard treatment for hypercalcemia of malignancy and because of the central role of osteoclasts in mediating bone disease, their role in the inhibition of osteolysis has been investigated.

5.2 Bone Pain

It has not been demonstrated convincingly that any of the currently available oral biphosphonates (etidronate, clodronate or pamidronate) can reduce metastatic bone pain. This was confirmed in a placebo-controlled study of oral clodronate in 55 patients with progressing bone metastases, mainly from breast cancer. Clodronate at 1600 mg/day significantly reduced bone pain, as assessed by a visual analogue scale, compared with an increase in bone pain in the placebo group, but did not reduce analgesic requirements (Robertson et al, 1995). When pooling the available data of several phase II trials with iterative intravenous pamidronate infusions, one-half of patients experienced relief of bone pain (Body et al, 1996).

However, these studies were not placebo controlled and the evaluation was sometimes open to criticism. Placebo-controlled studies have nevertheless confirmed that both clodronate and pamidronate exert significant analgesic effects (Ernst et al, 1992; Coleman et al, 1996). The analgesic activity of biphosphonates is useful for patients with advanced disease who are refractory to antineoplastic treatments. The optimal timing of biphosphonate administration in patients with painful bone metastases has not been clearly determined.

5.3 Osteolytic Process

Biphosphonates can lead to bone "recalcification" by themselves, although the clinical implications and benefit of these findings remain to be demonstrated (Body et al, 1996). Interestingly, preliminary reports of two large randomised clinical trials of pamidronate showed an increase in bone response rates to chemotherapy plus pamidronate (33%) compared to chemotherapy alone (18%) (Hortobagyi et al, 1996), although this effect was not seen with endocrine therapy (Theriault et al, 1996). The investigators used different therapeutic schedules in these trials. Biochemical markers of bone metabolism and turnover indicate that the dose of 90 mg pamidronate is the most adequate to inhibit bone resorption in this patient population (Body et al, 1995). Iterative biphosphonate infusions are therefore useful as an additional systemic treatment for lytic bone metastases. The prolonged administration of biphosphonates also decreases the complication rate of established bone metastases (Body et al, 1996).

5.4 Prevention of Complications of Bone Metastases in Patients with Breast Cancer

Many studies have reported a beneficial effect of oral biphosphonate treatment on the morbidity caused by bone metastases (Coleman et al, 1998; Morton et al, 1988; Thiebaud et al, 1991). Two large multicentre phase III trials in patients with breast cancer metastatic to the skeleton indicated that the prolonged administration of clodronate or pamidronate reduces the frequency of morbid skeletal events by 28 and 38%, respectively (Paterson et al, 1993; Van Holten-Verzantvoort et al, 1987, 1993).

The clodronate trial was a randomised, double-blind, placebo-controlled study, including 173 patients with bone metastases due to breast cancer. In the clodronate-treated group (1600 mg/day), there was a significant reduction in the total number of hypercalcaemic episodes, in the incidence of vertebral fractures and in the rate of vertebral deformity. Trends were seen in favour of clodronate for non-vertebral fracture rate and radiotherapy requirements for bone pain. In this large-scale trial, no significant survival differences were observed between the two groups.

In another large-scale, randomised, unblinded study, Van Holten-Verzantvoort et al (1987, 1993) reported that administration of daily oral pamidronate to breast cancer patients with bone metastases lowered the morbidity from skeletal metastases by about one-half. In the pamidronate-treated group, the incidence of hypercalcemia, bone pain and symptomatic imminent fractures was reduced by 65, 30 and 50% respectively. A significant decrease in the need for systemic treatment changes and radiotherapy by 35 and 33% was observed. Moreover, the authors could not detect significant effects on the skeletal event-free period, survival, or the radiological appearances of the lytic lesions. Dose-dependent efficacy was suggested, as larger effects were observed in patients who initially received 600 mg pamidronate daily compared to patients who received 300 mg daily throughout the study period (Van Holten-Verzantvoort et al, 1987, 1993).

The poor and variable absorption of the existing compounds, the requirement to take the drug a long time before or after food intake, the occasional intolerance superimposed on the frequent digestive complaints and lack of appetite of cancer patients, all make the intravenous route more attractive than the oral route in cancer patients with established bone metastases (Body et al, 1996).

Three randomised studies of regular intravenous pamidronate have been completed (Conte et al, 1994; Hortobagyi et al, 1996; Theriault et al, 1996). In the first pamidronate study, patients were randomised in a multicentre open trial comparing infusions of 45 mg pamidronate every 3 weeks plus chemotherapy or chemotherapy alone in 295 patients with lytic bone metastases from breast cancer. The authors reported an increase in median time to bone progression in the pamidronate group (249 days) compared to the control group (168 days). This slowing of bone destruction was accompanied by reductions in overall morbidity, as shown by significantly increased numbers of patients reporting marked pain relief, by trends in the improvement of other symptomatic variables, and by reduction in the incidence of complications of bone metastases. Nevertheless, the incidence of pain requiring radiotherapy was not significantly reduced by pamidronate, and there was no difference in survival between the two groups (Conte et al, 1994, 1996).

Double-blind, randomised, placebo-controlled trials have been conducted in a large series of breast cancer patients with lytic bone metastases (Hortobagyi et al, 1996; Theriault et al, 1996), comparing infusions of 90 mg pamidronate every 3–4 weeks for 1 year with placebo, in addition to chemotherapy or hormone therapy. The results were particularly impressive in the chemotherapy trial, which included 382 patients. The authors reported a significant reduction in the mean skeletal morbidity rate (number of skeletal-related events per year) in the pamidronate group compared to the control group. Moreover, there was a significant reduction in the number of non-vertebral pathological fractures, and in the proportion of patients having radiation or surgery to bone, in the pamidronate group.

Theriault et al (1996) recently presented a randomised controlled phase III evaluation of intravenous pamidronate used in association with hormonal therapy in 372 women with lytic bone metastases. The incidence of fracture or the need for radiation therapy was reduced by 25–30% in the pamidronate-treated patients, in whom there was also a decrease in pain scores from baseline. This report, as well as those by Robertson et al (1995), Hortobagyi et al (1996) and Paterson et al (1996), support the view that biphosphonates can reduce the morbidity from skeletal metastases in women being treated for metastatic breast cancer. The optimal therapeutic schedule for pamidronate is not known with certainty, but monthly infusions are clearly effective and this schedule, while not ideal, is compatible with palliation of advanced malignancy (Body et al, 1996).

5.5 Prevention of Bone Metastases Development in Patients with Breast Cancer

Trials in patients with established bone metastases suggest that long-term administration of biphosphonates could prevent or delay the development of bone metastases (Conte et al, 1994, 1996). Randomised, multinational, controlled, phase III trials in breast cancer patients with bone metastases compared 45 mg pamidronate infusions every 3 weeks in association with chemotherapy alone until progression of disease (Conte et al, 1994, 1996). The median time to progressive disease in bone was increased by 48% in patients who received pamidronate (249 vs 168 days). Convincing evidence of a delay in progression in skeletal disease was accompanied by reductions in overall morbidity, as shown by significantly increased numbers of patients reporting marked pain relief, by trends in the improvement of other symptomatic variables, and by reduction in the incidence of complications of bone metastases (Conte et al, 1996). The response rates of extraskeletal metastases and median survival were similar in the treatment groups.

Paterson et al (1996) reported the results of a randomised, double-blind, controlled study comparing oral clodronate (1600 mg/day) to placebo in addition to antitumour therapy in women with recurrent breast cancer in the absence of skeletal metastases. Fewer patients developed skeletal metastases during clodronate treatment and the total number of skeletal metastases was significantly decreased. The authors concluded that oral clodronate reduces the rate of progression of skeletal metastases in patients with recurrent breast cancer and provides a useful adjunct in the management of these patients. This is the one of the first clinical studies suggesting that an agent with an effect predominantly on normal tissue cells (osteoclasts) might influence the clinical appearance of metastatic disease. Trials in operable breast cancer are warranted and underway.

Diel et al (1997) recently presented the results of a prospective randomised study comparing oral clodronate (1600 mg/day) over 2 years with control patients in the adjuvant treatment of breast cancer patients. The bone relapse-free interval was longer (23 months) in the treatment group compared with the control group (16 months). This study showed that a reduction in the number and incidence of bone metastases is possible by adjuvant treatment with oral clodronate (administered over 2 years). Even non-bone metastases were reduced. However, the number of patients was limited (284) and follow-up was moderate (median of 36 months) (Diel et al, 1997). Prospective randomised studies should be performed to confirm these results.

5.6 Summary

Biphosphonates represent a major therapeutic advance in the management of tumour-induced osteolysis and skeletal morbidity, especially from breast cancer and multiple myeloma. They successfully treat hypercalcaemic episodes, relieve bone pain and may lead to recalcification of lytic metastases. Prolonged use of clodronate or pamidronate decreases the frequency of skeletal-related events in patients with metastatic bone disease. Another putative role for biphosphonate treatment is the prevention or delaying of the development of bone metastases in breast cancer patients. Pamidronate and clodronate are currently undergoing evaluation as preventive agents for prolonging bone metastasis-free survival in patients with extra-osseous metastases.

References

Body JJ (1992) Bone metastases and tumor-induced hypercalcemia. Curr Opin Oncol 4:624–631.

Body JJ, Dumon JC, Piccart M et al (1995) Intravenous pamidronate in patients with tumor induced osteolysis a biochemical dose-response study. J Bone Mineral Res 10:1191–1196.

Body JJ, Coleman RE, Piccart M (1996) Use of biphosphonates in cancer patients. Cancer Treatment Reviews 22:265–287.

Coleman RE, Woll PJ, Miles H et al (1998) Treatment of bone metastases from breast cancer with (3-amino-1-hydroxypropylidene)-1,1biphosphonate (APD). Br J Cancer 58:621–625.

Coleman RE, Vinholes J, Abbey ME (1996) Double-blind randomized trial of pamidronate for the palliative treatment of metastatic bone disease. Proc Am Soc Clin Oncol 15:528(Abstract 1506).

Conte PF, Giannessi PG, Latreille J et al (1994) Delayed progression of bone metastases with pamidronate therapy in breast cancer patients: a randomized, multicenter phase III trial. Ann Oncol 5(suppl 7):S41–44.

Conte PF, Latreille J, Mauriac F et al (1996) Delay in progression of bone metastases in breast cancer patients treated with intravenous pamidronate: results from a multinational randomized controlled trial. J Clin Oncol 14:2552–2559.

Diel IJ, Solomayer R, Goerner C et al (1997) Adjuvant treatment of breast cancer patients with the biphosphonate clodronate reduces incidence and number of bone and non-bone metastases. Proc Am Soc Clin Oncol 16:130a(Abstract).

Ernst DS, MacDonald RN, Paterson AHG et al (1992) A double-blind, cross-over trial of IV clodronate in metastatic bone pain. J Pain Symptomatol Management 7:4–11.

Hortobagyi GN, Theriault RL, Porter L et al (1996) Efficacy of pamidronate in reducing skeletal complications in patients with breast cancer and lytic bone metastases. N Engl J Med 335:1836–1837.

Hughes DE, Wright KR, Uy HL et al (1995) Biphosphonates promote apoptosis in murine osteoclasts in vitro and in vivo. J Bone Mineral Res 10:1478–1487.

Löwik CWGM, der Pluijm G, van der Wee-Pals et al (1988) Migration and phenotypic transformation of osteoclast precursors into mature osteoclasts: the effects of a biphosphonate. J Bone Mineral Res 2:185–192.

Morton AR, Canctrill JA, Pillar GV et al. (1988) Sclerosis of lytic bone metastases after disodium aminohydroxypropylidene biphosphonate (APD) in patients with breast carcinoma. Br Med J 297:772–773.

Paterson AHG, Powles TJ, Kanis JA et al (1993) Double-blind controlled trial of oral clodronate in patients with bone metastases from breast cancer. J Clin Oncol 11:59–65.

Paterson AHG, McCloskey EV, Ashley S et al (1996) Reduction of skeletal morbidity and prevention of bone marrow metastases with oral clodronate in women with recurrent breast cancer in the absence of skeletal metastases. Proc Am Soc Clin Oncol 15:104(Abstract).

Ralston SH (1992) Medical management of hypercalcemia. Br J Clin Pharmacol 34:11–20.

Reitsma PH, Teitelbaum SL, Bijvoet OL et al (1982) Differential action of the biphosphonates (3-amino-1-hydroxypropylene)-1,1-biphosphonate (ADP) and dosodium dichloromethylidene (Cl2MDP) on rat macrophage-mediated bone resorption in vitro. J Clin Invest 70:927–933.

Robertson AG, Reed NS, Ralston SH (1995) Effect of oral clodronate on metastatic bone pain: a double-blind, placebo-controlled study. J Clin Oncol 13:2127–2130.

Sahni M, Guenther HL, Fleisch H et al (1993) Biphosphonates act on rat bone resorption through the mediation of osteoblasts. J Clin Invest 91:2004–2011.

Theriault R, Lipton A, Leff R et al (1996) Reduction of skeletal complications in breast cancer patients with osteolytic bone metastases receiving hormone therapy by monthly pamidronate sodium (Aredia) infusion. Proc Am Soc Clin Oncol 15:122(Abstract).

Thiebaud D, Leyvraz S, von Fliedner V et al (1991) Treatment of bone metastases from breast cancer and myeloma with pamidronate. Eur J Cancer 27:37–41.

Van Holten-Verzantvoort ATM, Bijvoet OLM, Hermans J et al (1987) Reduced morbidity from skeletal metastases in breast cancer patients during long-term biphosphonate (APD) treatment. Lancet ii:983–985.

Van Holten-Verzantvoort ATM, Kroon HM, Bijvoet OLM et al (1993) Palliative pamidronate treatment in patients with bone metastases from breast cancer. J Clin Oncol 11:491–498.

6 Hormonal Therapy

M. Tubiana-Hulin and P. Soulié

6.1 Introduction

Bone lesions are the most common sites of metastasis for prostate and breast carcinoma, and may also occasionally result from endometrial carcinoma.

These tumour types arise in endocrine-dependent organs. Androgens are the physiological regulators of normal prostatic tissue, while oestrogens and progestins regulate growth and proliferation of normal breast and endometrium. Oestrogen exposure has a role in the pathogenesis of endometrial and breast carcinoma; tumour development and progression can also be influenced by the hormonal environment.

A logical approach to the treatment of these diseases is endocrine manipulation, which was implemented for the first time in antitumour therapy 100 years ago (Beatson, 1896); since then, indications for its use have increased considerably. Hormonal therapy is aimed at depriving tumours of hormonal stimuli by lowering either oestrogen or androgen levels or by competitively blocking their receptors. In the past three decades, endocrine therapy has evolved from being a suppressive surgical procedure (orchidectomy, oophorectomy, adrenalectomy, hypophysectomy) to include an expanding number of medical tools. New agents that are currently available (anti-oestrogens, anti-aromatases, luteinising hormone-releasing hormone (LH-RH) agonists) have an enlarged spectrum of activity, but also less toxicity. Reduction in tumour volume or inhibition of tumour growth can be consistently obtained and disease-related symptoms relieved in a significant number of treated patients. However, although endocrine therapy initially leads to objective clinical response or disease stabilisation, all tumours will eventually become resistant. Many patients (mainly with breast cancer) may respond sequentially to different hormonal manipulations but all will finally have hormone-independent disease.

6.2 Breast Cancer

6.2.1 Basis of Hormonal Therapy for Breast Cancer

6.2.1.1 Hormonal Factors in the Pathogenesis of Breast Cancer

Both oestrogens and progesterone play a major role in the pathogenesis of breast cancer, affecting the rate of proliferation of breast epithelial cells. Experimental in vivo data confirm this hypothesis (Henderson and Bernstein, 1996): exogenous oestrogens can increase the incidence of mammary tumours and the tumour yield in spontaneous or induced rodent mammary tumours, whereas ovariectomy or anti-oestrogenic therapy have the opposite effects. In humans, the possible influence of cumulative exposure to oestrogen or progesterone on breast cancer incidence was suggested by epidemiological studies, which isolated risk factors (early menarche, late menopause, obesity, diethylstilboestrol (DES) treatment, hormone replacement therapy) and protective factors (ovariectomy, early first pregnancy, lactation, physical activity), both reflecting hormonal influence. Some clinical studies have attempted to correlate breast cancer risk and oestrogen exposure by comparing oestradiol blood levels in patients with breast cancer with those in controls. In recent studies, breast cancer patients had significantly higher free oestradiol plasma levels than controls.

6.2.1.2 Mechanisms of Action

Oestrogen and progesterone exert their mitogenic effects through the binding and activation of specific nuclear receptors (Stein et al, 1995). Oestrogen and progesterone receptors belong to the superfamily of steroid receptors and are located predominantly in the nucleus of target cells. As progesterone receptors are normally induced by oestrogen, their presence reflects a functional endocrine response pathway.

When the oestrogen receptor protein binds to DNA, transcriptional activation of oestrogen-regulated genes is initiated, leading to the production, by the breast cancer cells, of various growth factors (epidermal growth factor, EGF; insulin growth factor, IGF_1; tissue growth factor, TGFa), which can stimulate tumour cell growth in both an autocrine and a paracrine manner. Receptors for EGF and IGF are found on breast cancer cells, binding respectively EGF, TGFa and IGF (Sutherland and Mobbs, 1995). A large amount of evidence indicates that oestrogen also controls a cascade of growth-regulating events potentially involved in tumour growth. Oestrogens are known to stimulate the synthesis of proteins involved in growth regulatory pathways such as myc, fos and jun, cyclins and cyclin-dependent kinases. In both normal and tumour tissue, the lack of such stimuli results in the triggering of apoptosis. Steroid deprivation can inhibit these stimulatory effects and endocrine responsiveness, i.e. tumour regression or stabilisation can occur in tumours where oestrogens play a central role in the control of cell growth.

6.2.1.3 *Steroid Receptor Status in Breast Cancer Tissue*

Postmenopausal patients are more likely to have oestrogen receptor-positive tumours than premenopausal women. In the former, about 65–80% of breast cancers have oestrogen receptors and 50–65% progesterone receptors.

The oestrogen and progesterone receptor status of breast cancer tissue from newly diagnosed primary tumours are a "standard" component of the prognostic factor checklist at the time of breast cancer diagnosis. The absence of both receptors predicts early relapse and poor survival. Receptor-negative tumours tend to have an aggressive histological grade and high proliferative rates, whereas receptor-positive tumours are more likely to have a differentiated phenotype and lower proliferative rates.

The steroid receptor status of primary tumours and metastases is a factor in deciding treatment options for metastatic breast cancer patients (Valavaara, 1997). Overall, first-line endocrine therapies can yield response rates of 30% in unselected patients (50% when including disease stabilisation). Data from large clinical studies have confirmed that knowledge of both oestrogen and progesterone receptor status improves the ability to predict the responsiveness to endocrine therapy. The presence of both oestrogen and progesterone receptors in primary tumours predicts high response rates to first-line hormonal manipulation (50–70%) in advanced breast cancer. When the receptor phenotype of the tumour is discordant (oestrogen receptor-positive and progesterone receptor-negative, or oestrogen receptor-negative and progesterone receptor-positive), the response rate to initial endocrine therapy is lower, ranging from 27 to 46%. Patients with tumours that express neither receptor have an 11% response rate to hormonal therapy. A quantitative correlation between the oestrogen receptor content of the tumour and response to treatment has also been demonstrated.

Overexpression of *her 2/neu* may also be a predictor of resistance to hormonal therapy in both oestrogen receptor-positive and -negative tumours (Honig, 1996).

Endocrine therapy studies have also isolated other well-defined factors associated with a greater likelihood of response to hormonal manipulation: menopausal status, older age, long interval from diagnosis to first recurrence, disease sites outside the viscera such as bone and soft tissue. These clinical indicators are still the basis of treatment decisions and will be discussed below.

6.2.1.4 *Sources of Oestrogens in Breast Cancer Patients*

Physiological sources of oestrogen differ according to menopausal status. Oestradiol, synthesised by the ovaries, is the major oestrogen in premenopausal women. Oophorectomy was the first form of endocrine therapy, described by Beatson in 1896. Ovarian ablation is still considered the treatment of choice for premenopausal patients with non-visceral metastatic disease. Suppression of the ovarian production of oestradiol can be achieved either by surgical or radiotherapeutic ablation or, more recently, by the use of LH-RH agonists.

After the menopause, the predominant form of oestrogen is oestrone and the major source of this oestrogen is peripheral aromatisation of adrenal androgen precursors. The peripheral tissues involved in this process are fat, muscle and the tumour itself. Adrenalectomy was used in selected patients during the late 1950s and 1960s to suppress oestrogen precursors in postmenopausal women.

Aromatase inhibitors were developed as an alternative to this surgical procedure and are now established as second-line treatments in this patient population.

In premenopausal patients, the plasma oestradiol concentration is similar to tumour tissue levels, whereas in postmenopausal women, the oestradiol content of breast cancer cells is 10–20 times greater than in plasma; this blood-tumour gradient suggests that the tumour itself is a site of oestrogen production. Blocking the steroid synthesis within the tumour may allow greater oestrogen deprivation and better tumour growth control. Aromatase inhibitors, especially new-generation ones with increased activity, can produce maximal inhibition.

6.2.2 Medical Agents as Endocrine Therapy for Advanced Breast Cancer

Oestrogen deprivation remains the goal of any endocrine therapy of breast cancer. Reduction of oestrogen exposure can be achieved either by ablation of hormone-producing glands or by adding agents that (1) inhibit the synthesis of oestrogen from androgen precursors (aromatase inhibitors), (2) block the oestrogen receptor (anti-oestrogens) or (3) suppress the pituitary production of gonadotrophins (LH-RH agonists, progestins).

In the past two decades, the trend has been to develop less invasive and toxic treatments (Honig, 1996). As a number of endocrine agents have become available, they have progressively replaced most ablative procedures (adrenalectomy, hypophysectomy), which are no longer indicated. Only ovarian ablation (either by surgery or radiation) still remains a valid therapeutic option in selected premenopausal women. The response rate to ovariectomy ranges from 21 to 37% in unselected patients.

More recently, new drugs with reduced side-effects and interesting spectra of activity (especially in patients who have failed tamoxifen treatment) have proven active and effective in controlled clinical trials and are already (or soon will be) commercially available (Howell et al, 1996). The hormonal agents currently used in clinical practice are reviewed here.

6.2.2.1 Anti-oestrogens

Tamoxifen is the hormonal agent that is most frequently used, both in the adjuvant setting and in metastatic breast cancer (Stein et al, 1995; Honig, 1996). This agent has gained wide acceptance since 1972, when randomised trials demonstrated that it was as active but less toxic than oestrogens or androgens.

Tamoxifen has also been accepted as an alternative to oophorectomy in premenopausal metastatic breast cancer patients.

Various mechanisms of tamoxifen action have been proposed; its effects are mediated primarily through the oestrogen receptor by competitive binding with oestrogens. Tamoxifen causes a significant decrease in circulating levels of IGF_1 and an increased synthesis of TGFa, both of which are oestrogen-receptor dependent. It also has partial oestrogen agonist properties, especially in the endometrium. Non-receptor-mediated effects are also described and may contribute to therapeutic activity. Tamoxifen inhibits protein kinase C; it antagonises calmodulin, which regulates many Ca^{2+}-dependent intracellular signalling pathways. Inhibition of angiogenesis, reduction of natural killer cell activity, as well as antioxidant effects have been reported more recently.

Tamoxifen has a biological half-life of approximately 7 days. At least 4 weeks of daily administration are necessary to achieve steady-state serum levels. A 6- to 12-week period is required to clear tamoxifen and its metabolites after cessation of treatment. The recommended dose is usually 20–40 mg, once daily.

The most common side-effects are nausea with occasional vomiting in 9% of patients, hot flushes in 8–15%, amenorrhoea in 16–38% and thrombophlebitis in 1–4%. Vaginal discharge, skin rash, dizziness and rare ocular disturbances, including night-time vision decrease, cataracts and retinopathy, have been described. Endometrial carcinoma is seen in about 1% of women who take the drug for periods of 5 years or longer. This long-term side-effect is not clinically relevant in the metastatic setting.

In about 1–3% of patients with skin lesions or bone metastases, the initiation of hormonal therapy with tamoxifen, oestrogens, progestins or androgens induces a tumour flare episode. This syndrome appears as worsening of bone pain, increased size and number of skin nodules and, rarely, hypercalcaemia. All these symptoms occur within the first 3 weeks of treatment initiation. In bone disease, it may indicate increased osteoblastic response with early healing; diffuse increase in uptake on bone scan, as well as concomitant elevation of alkaline phosphatase serum levels, support this hypothesis. Such reactions should be recognised for what they are and failure of tamoxifen should not be claimed prematurely.

As first-line therapy in metastatic breast cancer patients, tamoxifen produces complete and partial responses in 30–35% of unselected patients, with response duration ranging from 9 to 18 months in most studies. A further 20% experience disease stabilisation beyond 6 months.

All metastatic tumours responding to tamoxifen treatment will ultimately progress or recur. Many investigators have examined this phenomenon and several mechanisms have been proposed to explain acquired resistance to this therapy: (1) modification of the oestrogen receptor structure and function, including generation of receptor mutants and an increased role for autocrine and paracrine growth factors; (2) alteration in intracellular uptake and/or metabolism of tamoxifen.

Tumour regression or stabilisation following interruption of treatment with tamoxifen has been reported in about 10–30% of patients (Howell et al, 1992). Most withdrawal responses occur in patients whose tumour responded initially with a subsequent regrowth while on tamoxifen. These observations confirm that tamoxifen could act as an oestrogen agonist.

Increased application of tamoxifen in the adjuvant setting has led to the need for suitable second-line hormonal therapy for relapsing patients.

More recently, a series of new anti-oestrogens has been developed. Most are non-steroidal, and are based on the triphenylethylene ring structure of tamoxifen. They have greater affinity for the oestrogen receptor than tamoxifen, with the exception of toremifene, and less oestrogen agonist activity. As first-line therapy in metastatic breast cancer, toremifene activity appears to be very similar to tamoxifen. Droloxifen looks promising, with response rates of 44 and 47% in the two higher-dose arms (40 and 100 mg/day) of a large international phase II trial; its shorter half-life makes it particularly useful in alternative delivery schedules. Other new non-steroidal anti-oestrogens (idoxifen, TAT 59) are also in clinical development in patients with advanced metastatic breast cancer.

The most interesting new compounds in clinical trials are the pure anti-oestrogens. Clinical data are now available for the ICI 182, 780 compound and suggest that it is active against tamoxifen-resistant metastatic breast cancer. In a recent phase II study, Howell et al. (1966) observed partial response or stabilisation in

13 out of 19 patients who had failed tamoxifen. The median duration of response (including stabilisation) was 18 months. Further studies are warranted to confirm the potential advantage of this new agent, administered by monthly intramuscular injection (Howell et al, 1996).

6.2.2.2 Aromatase Inhibitors

Aromatase inhibitors are classified into two main groups. Type I inhibitors have an androgen structure and are referred to as steroidal inhibitors (formestane, exemestane), while type II inhibitors are azoles (aminoglutethimide, letrozole, vorozole, anastrozole) (Miller, 1997).

Until recently, aminoglutethimide was the only available representative of this family. This agent was first proposed for treatment of breast cancer patients in 1973, acting as a "medical adrenalectomy". It blocks steroid hydroxylation and cleavage enzymes, inducing deficient steroidogenesis. It increases adrenocorticotrophin (ACTH) by a feedback mechanism. Low-dose glucocorticoids (20–40 mg daily) must be administered to avoid symptoms of adrenal suppression and stimulation.

The efficacy of aminoglutethimide is similar to that of surgical adrenalectomy. In first-line hormonal therapy of metastatic breast cancer, clinical response rates in postmenopausal patients have been shown to be comparable to those of tamoxifen. Aminoglutethimide is effective as second-line therapy in patients who have previously responded to tamoxifen, with a 30% response rate. The interrelationship between these two hormonal agents is of interest, with tamoxifen being less frequently beneficial after the aromatase inhibitor. These data suggest that aminoglutethimide should follow rather than precede tamoxifen.

Common side-effects include lethargy in about 40% of patients, dizziness in 16% and nausea/vomiting in 10–15%. Most side-effects are observed within the first 2–4 weeks after initiation of treatment; they usually regress after 6 weeks. Another common toxicity observed in about one-third of patients is a transient morbilliform maculopapular skin rash. The recommended dose range is between 500 and 1000 mg daily, with gradually increasing doses; this schedule causes fewer soporific symptoms.

New generations of aromatase inhibitors, with greater selectivity and potency, have been developed recently.

Formestane (4-hydroxyandrostendione) is the first type I inhibitor commercially available. Because of extensive first-pass liver metabolism, intramuscular injections are preferred. In postmenopausal women who have failed prior tamoxifen or aminoglutethimide, the reported objective response rate is about 20%. Formestane was shown to be as effective as megestrol acetate in controlled trials and its toxicity profile compares favourably; side-effects of 4-hydroxyandrostenedione are mainly pain at the injection site and hot flushes.

Exemestane is a second-generation steroid inhibitor, given orally. Clinical evaluation of this agent is ongoing and interesting activity has been observed in postmenopausal patients, including aminoglutethimide-pretreated patients.

Four non-steroidal inhibitors have been developed (fadrozole, letrozole, vorozole, anastrozole); all have greater potency and specificity in inhibition of aromatases, with values 60–1000 times greater than that of aminoglutethimide in the placental microsome assay. In postmenopausal women, treatment with anastrozole reduces the percentage of aromatisation by 96–98% and suppresses plasma levels of oestrone, oestradiol and oestrone sulphate by 86.5, 83.5 and 93.5%, respectively. Fadrozole, vorozole and anastrozole are active after tamoxifen, with response rates in about 10–13% of patients and stabilisation in 24–50%.

Vorozole and anastrozole were at least as effective as megestrol acetate in randomised trials (Goss et al, 1997; Buzdar et al, 1996), whereas letrozole and vorozole have shown greater clinical benefit than aminoglutethimide (Marty et al, 1997; Bergh et al, 1997).

The major side-effects associated with these new aromatase inhibitors are mild nausea/vomiting, hot flushes and anorexia. Lack of weight gain make them more attractive than progestins for second-line therapy in patients failing tamoxifen.

6.2.2.3 *Progestins*

The two progesterone derivatives currently available for metastatic breast cancer treatment are medroxyprogesterone acetate and megestrol acetate. Various mechanisms of action have been postulated for these agents, including reduction of oestrogen receptor content, inhibition of pituitary gonadotrophin secretion, direct effects on tumour cells through the expressed progesterone receptors and increased oestrogen catabolism. Many trials have documented response rates of 25–45% in pretreated patients. Progestative agents are active in premenopausal women. In recent phase III studies, megestrol acetate produced objective response in about 12–18% of patients who had received prior tamoxifen. A controversy still exists regarding the dose-effect relationship for each drug. Discordant results have been reported from randomised trials, and an advantage for dose escalation remains unproven. Medroxyprogesterone acetate is administered either by intramuscular injections or orally (500–1000 mg daily). The standard daily dose for megestrol acetate is usually 160 mg. Reported side-effects are weight gain, fluid retention, vaginal bleeding, improved appetite and thromboembolic events, more frequently observed at high doses.

6.2.2.4 *LH-RH Agonists*

LH-RH analogues can induce a reversible medical castration. They are as effective as tamoxifen in premenopausal patients. When given alone in a postmenopausal population, response rates of about 10% were reported. Common side-effects include transient hot flushes and decreased libido.

6.2.2.5 *Androgens*

Various androgenic agents have been used in the past for the treatment of metastatic breast cancer. Response rates of about 20% have been reported. However, virilising side-effects have rendered these endocrine therapies undesirable.

6.2.2.6 Oestrogens

Oestrogens (DES, ethinyloestradiol) are effective therapies but are rarely used today because of their serious side-effects (nausea/vomiting, fluid retention, cardiovascular disorders).

6.2.2.7 Corticosteroids

Corticotherapy alone has limited antitumour activity in metastatic breast cancer patients. However, when added to tamoxifen or ovariectomy, corticosteroids have been reported to increase significantly response rate as well as overall survival in one controlled trial. They also provide good palliation, especially for bone pain and dyspnoea.

6.2.2.8 Antiprogestins

Two antiprogestins have entered the clinical development stage (mifepristone (RU 486) and onapristone). In first-line hormonal therapy, mifepristone showed a low response rate (9%), even in selected patients (progesterone receptor-positive tumours). Clinical development of onapristone has stopped because of liver toxicity. Newer analogues of this family are being developed (Howell et al, 1996).

6.2.3 Indications for and Choice of Hormonal Therapy in Metastatic Breast Cancer

6.2.3.1 Selection of Candidates for Hormonal Therapy

Metastatic breast cancer remains a lethal disease. The goal of any treatment is, in most cases, palliation. Currently available treatments (hormonal and chemotherapy) provide only temporary control of cancer growth. However, sequential use of these different therapies can extend the overall survival of patients and provide good quality of life. In the past two decades, the incorporation of several new cytotoxic/cytostatic agents, such as anthracyclines, anti-oestrogens and aromatase inhibitors, have contributed to this improvement.

Metastatic breast cancer is so heterogenous in its clinical course that any treatment decision should be tailored to the individual according to well-established predictive or prognostic factors.

Age, menopausal status, hormonal receptor level and clinical patterns of relapse, reflecting tumour indolence and invasion, are the main determinants in assessing each patient's prognosis. Among all available patient characteristics, tumour bulk, nature of disease sites as well as disease-free interval are the major factors to take into account in planning treatment. Disease extent should be evaluated by a complete physical examination, bone scan, chest radiograph, an abdominal computed tomography scan and plain radiographs of the involved bone segments. A complete blood count and routine chemistries, including transaminases, alkaline phosphatases and calcaemia, are also required.

Although the majority of patients will display osseous metastases during the course of the disease, only 15–20% present initially with lesions limited to bone. In the heterogeneous population of breast cancer patients, the clinical course of bone-dominant disease differs significantly from those with multivisceral presentation. Patients with exclusive bone disease have a better overall survival than those with visceral metastases (28 months vs 13 months). Osseous metastases occur later than visceral metastases and are more common in patients with well-differentiated primary tumours, likely to present a higher content of oestrogen receptor. All these characteristics are those classically predicting hormone dependence.

Disease-free interval (time from primary tumour treatment to first metastasis) is another important prognostic indication, as it reflects tumour aggressiveness. Finally, patients with limited, slowly growing soft tissue and/or bone lesions are more likely to have a better prognosis and hormone-dependent tumours.

As previously discussed, the hormone receptor content of the primary breast tumour is also a good predictor of efficacy of any hormonal manipulations: selection of patients with rich oestrogen receptor-positive tumours provides about 50% chance of response. Because of their favourable therapeutic index, hormonal agents are the systemic treatment of choice for these selected patients.

6.2.3.2 *Selection of Hormonal Therapy*

The choice of endocrine therapy depends on the patient's menopausal status, prior hormonal therapy (given in an adjuvant or metastatic setting) and the toxicity profile of the various treatments now available (Honig, 1996).

In premenopausal patients, the first hormonal treatment can be chosen from among tamoxifen, ovarian ablation or LH-RH agonists. In the postmenopausal population, tamoxifen is still the first-line therapy of choice. Until recently, progestins and aromatase inhibitors (mainly aminoglutethimide) were given as second-line hormonal therapy. In the future, the new aromatase inhibitors, which are less toxic, are likely to replace aminoglutethimide as well as progestins in this clinical situation, while their role as first-line treatment is being investigated.

Many patients with oestrogen receptor-positive tumours have previously received tamoxifen as adjuvant treatment for several years. At the time of relapse, second-line hormonal therapy should be decided according to the treatment-free interval and the clinical presentation of the metastatic disease.

6.2.3.3 *Time to Response*

Response to hormonal therapy tends to be gradual and an observation period of 23 months in the absence of clear signs of progression is necessary to avoid premature interruption of treatment. Tumour flare syndrome may also occur at the start of some hormonal therapies, especially in patients with bone metastases, and should be recognised as such.

6.2.3.4 *Salvage Therapy*

About half of patients who respond to first-line hormonal therapy would be expected to benefit from second-line therapy, while 20% of those who failed first-line hormonal therapy may respond to second-line (Stein et al, 1995). Disease stabilisation and symptom relief, as well as objective response, may also be observed in third-line therapy (Iverson et al, 1993). Initiation of chemotherapy should not be delayed for patients with diffuse bone lesions who progress rapidly on hormone therapy and require new effective systemic treatment. For these patients, bone lesion radiation therapy can be added to hormonal therapy to relieve focal pain and prevent pathological fractures. However, extensive radiation in multiple separate fields will significantly reduce bone marrow reserve and hamper haematological tolerance of any future chemotherapy.

6.2.3.5 Role of Combination Therapy

In the past, no hormonal agent combination has been clearly shown to induce survival advantage over sequential single-agent therapy, although combined treatment may produce higher response rates. More recently, the combination of LH-RH agonists with tamoxifen was reported to significantly improve antitumour efficacy as well as overall survival in premenopausal metastatic breast cancer patients, when compared with each drug alone (Klijn et al, 1996). Novel combination approaches are now being tested in clinical trials, including retinoids or somatostatin analogues. In vitro/in vivo synergistic effects with tamoxifen have been demonstrated with these agents.

Hormone therapy is a well-established systemic treatment option for carefully selected metastatic breast cancer patients, giving clinical response rates and response durations similar to the standard chemotherapy combinations. In 1997, commercially available agents provided a better tolerance of therapy for the majority of treated patients, as well as allowing new strategies to be tested in the future (new hormonal therapy combinations, alternative hormonal therapies).

6.3 Prostate Cancer

Hormonal therapy has been the main treatment of prostate cancer since the 1940s, when Huggins and Hodges demonstrated that about 80% of these cancers were hormone sensitive, and that gonadal androgen deprivation by castration or oral oestrogens resulted in tumour regression or stabilisation.

Unfortunately, responses are not durable and virtually all patients progress while receiving hormone therapy. Alternative hormonal therapies have been developed; however, none as yet has clearly demonstrated a survival gain. Non-hormonal treatments such as chemotherapy, chemohormonal therapy, radioactive isotopes and radiotherapy can also be used, but patient age and limited haematopoietic medullary reserves due to bone involvement mean that such approaches have limited tolerance.

6.3.1 Evaluation of Response to Treatment

Prostatic bone metastatic lesions, usually of osteoblastic or mixed type, are difficult to evaluate as no measurable target can be determined on imaging studies. Bone scintigraphy is a sensitive and rapid technique for detecting areas of bone involvement, and extension of skeletal involvement on radionuclide bone scans is of prognostic value (Yamashita et al, 1993); however, treatment-related modifications are difficult to interpret if the interval between two examinations is less than 4–6 months.

Serial determinations of prostate-specific antigen (PSA) level are sensitive and reliable indicators of advanced prostatic disease evolution and its response to treatment. Therapeutic response criteria based on this marker have been used in several multicentre international trials: a reduction of more than 50% of initial PSA level indicated response to treatment. Moreover, a reduction of 90% of pre-treatment PSA level could predict a longer time to progression and better outcome (Matzkin and Soloway, 1992); an increase in PSA levels after attaining a nadir indicates progression, as this phenomenon almost always precedes extension of high spots on bone scans and reappearance of bone pain (Newling et al, 1992).

In the rare cases of advanced prostatic cancer without an increase in serum PSA level, evaluation of response is based on serial bone scans and/or prostatic acid phosphatases. At very advanced stages of the disease, other measurable parameters such as anaemia or weight loss can be used.

6.3.2 Hormonal Treatment

"Classical" or standard first-line treatment of advanced prostatic cancer is based on the conclusions of the Veterans Administration Cooperative Urologic Research Group, which demonstrated the equivalence between surgical castration, oestrogens and the combination of these two treatments in stage D prostate cancer (Hanks et al, 1993). However, oestrogens are now avoided because of their cardiovascular side-effects.

During the past 20 years, research on hormonal treatment of prostatic cancer has followed two directions: to ameliorate tolerance in comparison with available standard therapies and to suppress androgenic stimuli totally in order to eliminate hormone-induced growth of prostatic tumour cells.

Ideally, the treatment must suppress testicular secretion, decrease adrenal androgenic secretion, prevent increase of prolactin, prevent formation of the dihydrotestosterone-androgenic receptor complex, and decrease a-reductase activity.

6.3.2.1 Castration

Surgical castration remains in widespread use. Subcapsular orchiectomy, preserving scrotal content, is psychologically better accepted than bilateral orchidectomy. This procedure was considered to be suboptimal because of the possibility of incomplete elimination of Leydig's cells. However, castrate testosterone levels and rapid disappearance of bone pain are achieved in most patients. Castration suppresses 90% of circulating androgens; 3 hours after surgery, testosterone level ranges between 10 and 50 ng/100 ml, whereas LH level rises. Disadvantages of surgical castration are the consequences of hypoandrogenia: impotence, sometimes mastodynia and hot flushes, but principally the irreversible nature of this procedure, which has no efficacy in 20% of patients.

6.3.2.2 *Gonadotrophin-Releasing Hormone Agonists*

Several agonist analogues of LH-RH have been available since the 1970s. The main modifications of the natural decapeptide are amino acid substitutions at residue 6 and addition of radical ethylamide and azaglycinamide at residue 10. These synthetic compounds, unlike the natural molecule, resist degradation by pituitary peptidases. Given at high doses, they saturate the LH-RH pituitary receptors, which are rendered insensitive to further stimulation. Administration of these compounds leads to an initial increase in LH, follicle-stimulating hormone (FSH) and testosterone, followed by a decrease in gonadotrophins, which become undetectable after 2–6 weeks, with a concomitant fall in gonadal steroid levels. Testosterone plasma levels decrease to castrate levels and remain stable as long as regular injections are repeated. Several depot preparations of gonadotrophin-releasing hormone agonists are used in Europe (leuprorelin, buserelin, goserelin and triptorelin). They can be given once every 28 days, 2 months or 3 months, depending on the slow-release formulation.

Clinical improvement usually appears 2 weeks after the first injection. Some patients may experience a transitory exacerbation of symptoms: increased bone pain, and, in rare cases, spinal cord compression and even rapid deterioration, followed by death. This tumour flare is related to an initial increase in gonadotrophins and appears within the first week of treatment. It must be prevented, especially in patients with extensive advanced disease with multivisceral involvement. Corticosteroids, oestrogens or anti-androgens administered a few days before agonist injection and continued during the first month can prevent this serious complication. Initial reports on the activity of gonadotrophin-releasing hormone agonists showed an equivalent rate of response duration and survival as in DES-treated patients, with significantly less cardiovascular toxicity (Osborne et al, 1990).

Furthermore, while clinical activity and hypoandrogenic side-effects are equivalent to castration (Vogelzang et al, 1995), they are reversible when treatment is discontinued.

6.3.2.3 *Anti-androgens*

Steroid anti-androgens: Cyproterone acetate and megestrol acetate are steroid compounds with progestational activity. They compete with dihydrotestosterone binding in the tumour androgen-steroid receptor complex, while decreasing gonadal androgen synthesis is a consequence of decrease in LH and FSH levels. They also partially inhibit 5a-reductase, while having intrinsic androgenic activity.

Cyproterone acetate is given in daily doses of 100–300 mg. As a first-line hormonal treatment, local response, progression rates and overall survival are equivalent to 3 mg DES, with less side-effects; however, fluid retention, thromboembolism and myocardial infarction have also been reported, and impotence, libido decrease and gynaecomastia are frequent (Robson and Dawson, 1996).

Megestrol acetate is less active than cyproterone acetate. Low doses of oestrogen (0.1 mg DES daily) have been used in combination with megestrol acetate to produce more effective pituitary suppression and reinforce clinical activity. However, side-effects are frequently observed.

Pure anti-androgens: Non-steroidal anti-androgens block the hypothalamo-pituitary androgen receptor, resulting in a secondary rise in gonadotrophin and testosterone levels.

Flutamide is transformed into several metabolites, hydroxyflutamide being responsible for the activity of the drug. It is administered three times daily for a total dose of 750 mg. Its side-effects differ from those of steroid anti-androgens; no cardiovascular or glucocorticoid-like effects are observed, and it has little effect on potency, libido or sperm count. Other side-effects are observed, however, such as gynaecomastia, gastrointestinal disturbances, and, rarely, hepatotoxicity. Flutamide and androgen suppression appear to have comparable activity when given as first-line treatment of advanced disease, but so far clinical trials have been too small to allow firm conclusions.

Nilutamide (Anandron) is a synthetic imidazole compound, with a prolonged half-life (approximately 2 days) that allows daily administration. The daily dosage is 300 mg initially, then 150 mg as a maintenance therapy. Side-effects are gynaecomastia, hot flushes, quite frequent ophthalmological side-effects (delay in accommodation to darkness), and rare cases of interstitial pneumonitis, but impotence is unusual (Decensi et al, 1991).

Bicalutamide (Casodex) is a new pure anti-androgen that can be administered once daily. It has little effect on hypothalamo-pituitary gonadotrophin secretion. It may be more effective than flutamide as second-line hormonal therapy (Robson and Dawson, 1996).

6.3.2.4 Combined Total Androgen Blockade

The androgen blockade concept was proposed by Labrie in the 1980s (Labrie et al, 1993). Its rationale is based on the fact that 5–10% of circulating androgens are produced by the adrenal gland. Such production persists despite castration and could enhance hypersensitive cellular clones, leading to early tumour escape. Therefore, total suppression of androgen sources would reduce the probability of regrowth of tumour cellular clones and prolong response duration. Several controlled clinical trials have tested this hypothesis, with a meta-analysis being available. Most studies compared surgical or medical castration + placebo with castration + anti-androgen (flutamide or nilutamide). Globally, they showed that immediate combined androgen blockade was superior to the delayed addition of an anti-androgen on progression: decrease in bone pain, improvement in objective response criteria of the National Prostatic Cancer Project and a more frequent normalisation of PSA were observed with the combination. However, the 1995 meta-analysis by the Prostate Cancer Trialists' Collaborative Group failed to demonstrate an improvement for median overall survival.

6.3.2.5 Oestrogens

High-dose oestrogens suppress testicular androgens as a consequence of pituitary gonadotrophin decrease; they also directly inhibit 5a-reductase activity. Suppression of the hypothalamic-pituitary axis is established within 10–14 days and persists as long as treatment is maintained. It induces a progressive testicular atrophy, and testicular androgen production remains very low for a long time after treatment is discontinued. A daily dose of less than 5 mg DES is recommended to limit non-hormonal side-effects; 3 mg daily is sufficient to suppress androgen testicular secretion, but serious side-effects are still observed: fluid retention, thrombophlebitis, heart failure and myocardial infarction. Tolerance problems also include nausea/vomiting and symptoms of hypoandrogenia. Gynaecomastia can be prevented by external radiotherapy to the breasts, delivering 8–10 Gy in one session. A daily dose of 1 mg DES is better tolerated and appears to be equivalent for antitumour clinical response. The low cost of this therapy is to be emphasised.

6.3.2.6 *Fosfestrol*

Diethylstilboestrol diphosphate is a water-soluble oestrogen that can be given intravenously in high doses. The drug is activated in the prostatic tissue, delivering oestrogen locally with little systemic exposure. Daily intravenous doses of 250–500 mg are given initially, with oral daily doses of 100–300 mg serving as maintenance. The response rate is low because this drug is usually administered as second-line therapy after escape from first-line hormonal treatment: objective responses are rare, but a decrease in bone pain and a temporary reduction in PSA level are consistently reported (Droz et al, 1993). Tolerance is acceptable; however, gynaecomastia, oedema and cardiovascular events have been reported in 5% of patients.

6.3.2.7 *Aminoglutethimide*

Aminoglutethimide blocks adrenal steroid biosynthesis by inhibiting 20,22- desmolase, several adrenocortical steroid hydroxylation enzymes, and the aromatases interfering in oestrogen synthesis. This latter activity has been utilised to treat advanced breast cancer. Decrease in cortisol levels must be compensated by simultaneous hydrocortisone administration to prevent adrenal insufficiency and to block the ACTH rise. Surgical adrenalectomy carried out in the past induced a clinical response in approximately 30% of selected patients with advanced prostatic cancer who had not responded to first-line hormonal treatment. A National Prostatic Cancer Project trial showed only a 10% objective partial response and 39% of short stabilisations. Side-effects include asthenia, dizziness and gastrointestinal disturbances, which are poorly tolerated in this group of patients.

6.3.2.8 *Ketoconazole*

Ketoconazole is an imidazole compound used to treat several fungal diseases. Given in high doses (1200 mg daily), it induces a durable inhibition of gonadal androgen biosynthesis, and a partial inhibition of adrenal steroids, with reduction in cortisol response to ACTH. Given as a first-line treatment, bone pain is reduced in 90% of cases. As a second-line treatment after castration, objective responses were seen in less than 15% of cases, while a temporary reduction in biological markers was seen in 50% of cases. Tolerance is fair, with gastrointestinal disturbances, hypoandrogenic symptoms and liver dysfunction, which can lead to hepatic toxic death in rare cases.

6.3.2.9 *Liorozole*

Liorozole is another imidazole derivative. Objective partial responses have been reported; its activity and toxicity are still being evaluated.

6.3.3 Indications

Advanced prostatic cancer patients with bone involvement should receive as first-line systemic treatment at least surgical or medical castration or, probably better, total androgen blockade. Anti-androgens alone are an option for younger patients who want to preserve their potency (Soloway and Matzkin, 1993).

All patients with advanced prostatic cancer eventually develop progressive hormone-insensitive disease when treated with androgen deprivation. Usually, a progressive increase in PSA levels precedes the reappearance of clinical symptoms, particularly bone pain or modifications on imaging studies. This escape phenomenon may be related to several mechanisms: (1) adaptation of hormone-sensitive cells, allowing regrowth in the presence of very low androgen concentrations; (2) growth of hormone-insensitive clones present before treatment in a phenotypically heterogenous tumour; (3) acquired conversion of previously androgen-sensitive cells into androgen-insensitive cells, related to genetic instability and clonal selection.

Results of second-line hormonal treatment in advanced prostate cancer are dependent on the mechanism of tumour resistance and on the type of first-line hormonal treatment. After castration alone, anti-androgens, adrenal androgen deprivation by any active agent or oestrogens can induce objective responses in less than 20% of patients. After failing anti-androgens alone, surgical or medical castration is often effective. On the other hand, after combined androgen blockade, response to second-line hormonal treatment is seldom objective and usually of short duration. An anti-androgen withdrawal syndrome was described by Kelley and Scher (1993), who reported a significant decrease in serum PSA level, sometimes associated with clinical improvement, when anti-androgen (flutamide) was discontinued in patients refractory to combined androgen blockade. This withdrawal syndrome had also been reported with other anti-androgens and megestrol acetate. This possibility should be tested in every patient with progression of their prostate cancer while on combined androgen blockade, before administration of another treatment, especially in those undergoing clinical trials (Small and Vogelzang, 1997).

6.4 Endometrial Cancer

Endometrial adenocarcinoma is the third most common hormone-responsive tumour, originating from hormonally regulated epithelium. Excessive endogenous oestrogen stimulation, as well as exogenous oestrogen exposure (including the partial agonist tamoxifen), have been implicated in the development of endometrial cancer. Hormonal receptors (oestrogen and progesterone receptors) have been identified in tumour tissue samples. Progesterone receptors are predominantly expressed, mainly in well-differentiated tumours.

Hormonal agents are of value in the management of selected patients with recurrent or advanced endometrial adenocarcinoma (Neijt, 1993). Recent studies have reported response rates of about 15% to progestins. In receptor-positive patients, higher activity has been observed, ranging from 40 to 60%. Unfortunately, most patients with stage IV tumours have poorly differentiated, receptor-negative disease. Tamoxifen is also active, with response rates of about 22%, even in patients who failed prior progestins. More recently, LH-RH agonists have been shown to have a significant antitumour effect (35% response rate) in recurrent endometrial adenocarcinoma.

References

Bergh J, Bonneterre J, Illiger HJ et al (1997) Vorozole (Rivizor) versus aminoglutethimide (AG) in the treatment of postmenopausal breast cancer relapsing after tamoxifen. Proc Asco 16:155a.

Buzdar A, Jonat W, Howell A et al (1996). Anastrazole, a potent and selective aromatase inhibitor, versus megestrol acetate in postmenopausal women with advanced breast cancer: results of overview analysis of two phase III trials. J Clin Oncol 14:2000–2011.

Decensi AU, Boccardo F, Guarneri D et al (1991). Monotherapy with nilutamide, a pure non-steroidal antiandrogen in untreated patients with metastatic carcinoma of the prostate. The Italian prostatic cancer project. J Urol 146:377–381.

Droz JP, Kattan J, Bonnay M et al (1993). High dose continuous infusion Fosfestrol in hormone resistant prostate cancer. Cancer 71:1123–1130.

Goss P, Wine E, Tannock I et al (1997). Vorozole versus Megace in postmenopausal women with metastatic breast carcinoma who had relapsed following tamoxifen. Proc Asco 16:155a.

Hanks GE, Myers CE, Scardino PT (1993) Cancer of the prostate. In: de Vita S, Hellman SA, Rosenberg JB (eds) Cancer: principles and practice of oncology. JB Lippincott, Philadelphia, pp 1073–1113.

Henderson BE, Bernstein L (1996) Endogenous and exogenous hormonal factors. In: Harris JR, Morrow M, Lippman ME et al (eds) Diseases of the breast. Lippincott-Raven, Philadelphia, New York, pp 185–200.

Honig SF (1996) Hormonal therapy and chemotherapy. In: Harris JR, Morrow M, Lippman ME et al (eds) Diseases of the breast. Lippincott-Raven, Philadelphia, New York, pp 185–200.

Horwich A, Waxman J, Schroder (1995) Tumours of the prostate. In: Peckham M, Pinedo HM, Veronesi U (eds) Oxford textbook of oncology, pp 1498–1530.

Howell A, Dodwell DJ, Anderson H et al (1992) Original article: response after withdrawal of tamoxifen and progestogens in advanced breast cancer. Ann Oncol 3:611–617.

Howell A, Downey S, Anderson E (1996) New endocrine therapies for breast cancer. Eur J Cancer 32A(4):576–588.

Iverson TJ, Ahern J, Smith IE (1993) Response to third-line endocrine treatment for advanced breast cancer. Eur J Cancer 29A(4):572–574.

Kelley WK, Scher HI (1993) Prostate specific antigen declines after antiandrogen withdrawal: the flutamide withdrawal syndrome. J Urol 149:607–609.

Klijn JGM, Seynaeve C, Beex L et al (1996) Combined treatment with buserelin (LHRH-A) and tamoxifen (TAM) vs single treatment with each drug alone in premenopausal metastatic breast cancer: preliminary results of EORTC study 10881. Proc Asco Abstract 132.

Labde F, Bellanger A, Simard J et al (1993) Combination therapy for prostate cancer: endocrine and biologic basis of its choice as new standard first line therapy. Cancer 71:1059–1067.

Marty M, Gershanovich M, Campos B et al (1997) Superior to aminoglutethimide (AG) in postmenopausal women with advanced breast cancer (ABC) previously treated with anti-estrogens. Proc Asco 16:156a.

Matzkin H, Soloway MS (1992) Response to second-line hormonal manipulation monitored by serum PSA in stage D2 prostate carcinoma. Urology 40(1):78–80.

Miller WR (1997) New drugs: aromatase inhibitors and breast cancer. Cancer Treat Rev 23:171–187.

Neijt JP (1993) Systemic treatment in disseminated endometrial cancer. Eur J Cancer 29A(4):628–632.

Newling DWW, McLeod D, Soloway M et al (1992) Distant disease. Cancer 70(1):365–367.

Osborne DR, Moffat LEF, Rees DLP et al (1990) A comparison of Zoladex, cyproterone acetate and stilbestrol in the treatment of patients with advanced prostate carcinoma. In: Murphy, Khoury, Chatelain et al (eds). Recent advances in urological cancers. Diagnosis and treatment. Paris, pp 53–55.

Prostate Cancer Trialists' Collaborative Group (1995) Maximum androgen blockade in advanced prostate cancer: an overview of 22 randomised trials with 3283 deaths in 5710 patients. Lancet 346:265–269.

Robson M, Dawson M (1996) How is androgen-dependent metastatic prostate cancer best treated? Hematol/Oncol Clin North Am 3:727–747.

Small EJ, Vogeizang NJ (1997) Second-line hormonal therapy for advanced prostate cancer: a shifting paradigm. J Clin Oncol 15(1):382–388.

Soloway MS, Matzkin H (1993) Antiandrogenic agents as monotherapy in advanced prostatic carcinoma. Cancer 71:1083–1088.

Stein RC, Coombes RC, Howell A (1995) The basis of hormonal therapy of cancer. In: Peckham M, Pinedo H, Veronesi U (eds) Oxford textbook of oncology, vol 1, sect 1–7, pp 629–648.

Sutherland DJ, Mobbs BG (1995) Hormones and cancer. In: Tannock IF, Hill RP (eds) The basic science of oncology, 2nd edn. McGraw-Hill, New York, pp 207–232.

Valavaara R (1997) Reliability of estrogen receptors in predicting response to antiestrogens. Oncology 11,5(suppl 4):14–18.

Vogelzang NJ, Chodak GW, Soloway MS et al (1995). Goserelin versus orchiectomy in the treatment of advanced prostate cancer: final results of a randomized trial. Urology 46(2):220–226.

Yamashita K, Denno K, Ueda T et al (1993) Prognostic significance of bone metastases in patients with metastatic prostate cancer. Cancer 71(4):1297–1302.

7 Cement-Containing Antimitotics

Ph. Hernigou

Buchholz and Hengelbrecht were the first to use cement as a vehicle for active drug substances when, in 1970, they combined gentamicin with Palacos cement. This combination with gentamicin was found to be stable and able to provide effective antibiotic activity against the main pathogens encountered in bone surgery.

On the basis of this example (Graham, 1978), it was possible to envisage using cement/drug mixtures to treat other orthopaedic complaints calling simultaneously for mechanical consolidation of the bone and in-situ release of a drug. One example would be the strengthening of bone with cement after resection of a bone tumour plus the local release of antimitotic drugs from the implant.

There are two causes of failure in the surgical treatment of metastatic tumours: first, local recurrence of the tumour is not always prevented, even after extratumoural surgical exeresis and systemic chemotherapy, and secondly, failure of osteosynthesis after surgery. For these reasons, we thought that it would be helpful to provide local chemotherapy (Hernigou et al, 1987–1993) during and immediately after surgery, for instance, by adding an antimitotic to the acrylic cement used to replace the bone loss or to seal reconstruction prostheses. It was thought that the antimitotic would be released into the surrounding tissues in the same way as many antibiotics (Hoff et al, 1981).

Cement was the first vehicle to be studied for the purpose of releasing local chemotherapy. Methyl polymethacrylate (PMMA) fulfils the two following criteria:

- It has good biocompatibility, which is necessary as the system has to remain in situ throughout the rest of the patient's life
- It is not biodegradable, so that it provides mechanical support for bone that has been weakened by the surgical exeresis of a neoplastic site.

Methotrexate was the first antimitotic to be tested for use in this way (because an antidote was available); subsequently, cisplatin and adriamycin have been reported to be released from acrylic cement. Other diffusion vehicles have also been described, such as hydroxyapatite, which could be suitable for local chemotherapy.

7.1 Study of the Release of Methotrexate

The first study investigated the in-vitro release of antimitotics included in acrylic cement. After confirming that this release does actually occur, starts rapidly and is maintained over a prolonged period, two further studies were carried out in vivo.

The second study was in dogs with spontaneous osteosarcoma, to investigate the release of the antimitotic from the cement into the plasma, systemic safety and the local activity of the antimitotic-loaded cement following exeresis of the neoplasm.

The third study was conducted in laboratory rats with implanted osteosarcomas. This type of tumour was used so that a large number of animals with tumours could be studied and divided into uniform groups. Under these experimental conditions, it was possible to monitor the progress of the tumours left in situ, as well as the histopathological changes brought about by the local action of antimitotics released from implants.

7.1.1 Kinetic Profile of the Release of Methotrexate from Implants

The release profiles from implants containing 1% w/w have shown that methotrexate is released more rapidly during the first 2 hours and 10% of the load is released within the first 18 hours. The rate of release then slows. Implants immersed in an extraction medium, which is changed regularly, continue to release methotrexate for 6 months, the quantities released initially being higher the greater the initial load.

7.1.2 Release of Methotrexate from Acrylic Cement

This has been investigated in vivo in dogs with spontaneous sarcoma. The loss of substance resulting from the exeresis of the tumour was compensated using freshly prepared methotrexate-loaded cement. The dose of methotrexate received ranged from 1.6 to 16 mg/kg. Two hours after being implanted, plasma levels of methotrexate ranged from 0.08 to 0.02 micromoles/litre (1 micromole of methotrexate = 0.455 mg). After 24 hours, the plasma levels were between 0.1 and 0.02 micromoles/litre and by the third day were no longer detectable. Toxic effects were observed on day 4 in the three animals that had received a dose of more than 200 mg methotrexate. The other animals, which had received a dose of between 100 and 150 mg, did not display any signs of toxicity. The survival curve of the animals in this group seemed to be better than that of the animals that underwent surgery without adjuvant treatment, where 85% of the animals had died within 7 months.

7.1.3 Efficacy of Methotrexate-Loaded Implants

This was investigated using the experimental model of osteosarcoma in the rat (Klein et al, 1977). Using implants equivalent to 1.5 mg of active constituent, tumour growth was temporarily slowed and the survival time of the animals significantly prolonged.

These experiments have shown that the rise in temperature that accompanies the polymerisation of the cement does not destroy methotrexate and, like antibiotics, methotrexate can be released from the cement.

Migration probably occurs as a result of diffusion; the cement constitutes a network of pores and microfissures, which makes it accessible to the liquid medium in which it is immersed. This liquid penetrates into the system and dissolves the crystals of methotrexate, which then diffuse into the surrounding medium. This mechanism is certainly the dominant one at work during the early stages of methotrexate release. It probably accounts for the initial peak that characterises the kinetics of methotrexate release.

It is logical to suppose that the outer layers of the cement are more accessible to the liquid medium than the inner layers.

7.2 Study of the Release of Cisplatin

Cisplatin, an antimitotic that is suitable for mixing with cement, is often used to treat primary bone tumours. In the context of bone metastases from visceral tumours, it is generally used in multiple-drug therapy of tumours that are characterised particularly by being resistant to radiotherapy and to other antimitotics: hence the appeal of a local cisplatin-based therapy, which has the advantage of being radio-sensitising.

Cisplatin takes the form of a whitish-yellow crystalline powder. It has no melting point as it decomposes without melting at 270°C. Cisplatin has a solubility in water at room temperature of 1 mg/ml.

In the solid state, cisplatin is relatively stable. In contrast, in solution it forms mono-aquo and di-aquo derivatives by the successive shedding of chloride ions. Cisplatin is most stable in solution at an acid pH and in the presence of chloride ions, which prevent a shift in the reaction equilibrium towards the formation of degradation products.

The mixture was prepared as follows: during the first step, the active constituent, cisplatin, was mixed with the polymer. A predetermined weight of polymer was placed in a porcelain mortar. A known quantity of cisplatin was then added in small fractions. In the second step, the monomer was added, depending on the quantity of polymer taken, the volume of polymer being that recommended by the manufacturer. The constituents were then thoroughly mixed for 4 minutes to form a homogeneous paste.

This paste was then poured into the barrel of a stoppered syringe. The mixture was then expelled by the pressure of the piston into polyethylene moulds measuring 6.7 mm (inside diameter) by 10.3 mm in height (cylindrical mould, Prolabo, Paris). The implants were left in the moulds for 24 hours, to allow complete polymerisation to take place, and then tipped out and kept in darkness at room temperature. The in-vitro release of cisplatin was investigated by placing the implants in a release medium with the following composition: sodium chloride 9 g; distilled water, q.s.p. (quantity sufficient provided) 1000 ml; 1 N hydrochloric acid, q.s.p. pH 4. After weighing, the implants were placed in the release medium at 37°C and stirred in darkness. Samples were taken at regular intervals and an equal volume of fresh medium was added to replace the reaction mixture removed. "Sink" conditions were maintained, i.e. the concentration of cisplatin in the release medium was never more than one-tenth of the saturation concentration (i.e. 100 mg cisplatin per litre).

The in-vitro release data obtained from implants containing various loads of cisplatin (from 1 to 20% w/w) are shown as a function of time: the quantities released were related to the initial concentration of cisplatin in the implants. For instance, after 90 days, the implants with the highest load had released about 12% of cisplatin, whereas implants containing 1% had released only 3% under these experimental conditions. It should also be noted that the release was incomplete from all the implants and never reached 100% of the initial load.

7.3 Diffusion Mechanism of Antimitotics

Studies of the release of antimitotics have concentrated on cisplatin. The release of cisplatin from implants initially involves the fraction of active substance in direct contact with the release medium. The remaining cisplatin then has to cross the polymer before it can be released. Methyl polymethacrylate acts as a barrier to the diffusion of the active substance. The principle underlying the investigation of the permeability of polymer films is to plot the time course of the quantity released from a given film of specific thickness.

Diffusion tests were carried out using a Plexiglas cell consisting of two compartments, between which the test film was inserted. The donor compartment contained a 1 mg/ml solution of cisplatin in acidified physiological saline at pH 4; the receiver compartment contained the same solution, but without the cisplatin. The volume of both compartments was 50 ml and the area of the film in contact with them was 12.566 cm^2. The cell was immersed in a thermostatically controlled water bath at 37°C. Two pumps ensured a closed-circuit circulation of both media with a flow rate of 5 ml/min.

The results were interpreted using Fick's laws of diffusion. According to this law, it is assumed that the coefficient of diffusion is independent of the concentration and the diffusion takes place in one direction only. The diffusion experiments have shown that in solution, cisplatin cannot cross a block of PMMA cement. Similarly, in the case of films, diffusion experiments have shown that cisplatin crosses the membrane with difficulty. Diffusion within the cement differed for two different types of film prepared: PMMA/MMA film and pure PMMA film. The former consists of preformed spheres of PMMA, linked to each other by adding monomer. The latter consists of PMMA alone, but its structure is no longer conserved as the polymer has previously been dissolved in dichloromethane (preparation of pure PMMA films).

In the case of pure PMMA films, diffusion experiments have shown that cisplatin in solution had great difficulty in crossing even a thin membrane. Cisplatin therefore appears to be unable to cross pure PMMA. In the case of PMMA/MMA films, we found that up to a certain thickness, cisplatin was readily able to diffuse across the membrane. This diffusion can be accounted for by the structure of the polymer, which is not a uniform matrix, but a layer of spheres of PMMA, which are linked to one another by the polymerised monomer. In solution, cisplatin must be able to diffuse into the relatively less compact zone between the spheres, which may have defects of structure and cohesion. However, at thicknesses from 133 microns, diffusion is slower, as if a thicker layer of spheres impedes the diffusion of the active constituent. These findings should be interpreted in the light of the structure of the cement viewed under electron microscopy, which reveals areas of regular polymer and defects, fissures that doubtless permit the diffusion of cisplatin.

It should be noted that the release is increased at higher concentrations of cisplatin: as a whole, the findings suggest a release mechanism involving a process of percolation. It is only above a certain load that the crystals of cisplatin are sufficiently numerous to constitute a continuous network within the matrix. As the external medium dissolves the outermost crystals, it is able to penetrate to the crystals deeper down, and so on.

7.4 Clinical Experience

The clinical research was done at the Henri Mondor hospital and has confirmed the experimental data obtained in animal studies. It provided the basis of the protocol for clinical use.

It is now possible to use the acrylic surgical cement used to reconstruct loss of bone tissue as a diffusion vehicle for local chemotherapy.

We are not reporting a clinical trial, nor discussing the possible advantages and disadvantages of such a form of local chemotherapy for the patient. However, it is of interest to report here the follow-up of patients who had undergone surgical operations during which an acrylic cement containing pharmacological concentrations of methotrexate was implanted. The data reported consisted of the plasma concentration of methotrexate, the urinary concentration and the concentration in the drain fluid.

During surgery, a dose of 100 mg methotrexate mixed with a complete dose of cement (46 g of polymer and 20 ml of monomer) was administered, followed by intramuscular administration of folinic acid between 72 and 86 hours later. This was well tolerated by the patients. The local concentration of methotrexate found in the drains within the first few hours reached levels 10,000 times greater than the plasma concentration and remained 100 times greater than the plasma concentration for the next 3 days if the drain was kept in place. Systemic distribution of this local chemotherapy was observed. The release and diffusion of methotrexate from the cement was continued well beyond 10 days (when methotrexate could still be assayed in one patient), since urinary excretion continued for at least 3 weeks.

It is difficult to compare the effect of a single administration of a dose that is continuously diffused (from the cement) with that of conventional chemotherapy administered sequentially by the intravenous route. The toxicity of phase-dependent agents (such as methotrexate) is known to be related to the length of time for which a lethal concentration is maintained for the cells in their sensitive phase. It is thought that, in the case of methotrexate, if no antidote is administered, there is no need to maintain a concentration of 0.05 micromoles per litre for more than 48 hours in man, and that a concentration of 0.01 micromoles is the efficacy threshold of the drug. It therefore appears to be prudent to monitor the change in plasma concentration of methotrexate even after this local chemotherapy. If the concentration remains too high on days 3 or 4, it is advisable to administer folinic acid for 24 hours. This has the effect of counteracting the general toxicity of this chemotherapy.

In a clinical study of cisplatin, which has a lower rate of diffusion from the cement than methotrexate, a dose of 200 mg cisplatin mixed with one packet of cement was used without any postoperative adverse haematological or renal effects being observed.

7.5 Conclusion

Hitherto, the peroperative chemotherapies available were regional and restricted to a given anatomical region by the following methods: extra-arterial infusion, infusion using a tourniquet, extra-corporeal circulation. These methods have given encouraging results, but complications have been reported, sometimes even amputation. If further developments in the investigations (Janmin Li, 1989) we have initiated confirm these early findings, this method of local neoplastic chemotherapy could offer an adjuvant therapy (Langendorff, 1989) that is likely to be easier to handle. There is no question that this therapy could offer a substitute for systemic chemotherapy (Rosen et al, 1982) or radiotherapy when these therapies are indicated.

References

Bucholz HW, Englebucht H (1970) Über die Depotwirkung einiger antibiotika bei vermischung mit dem kunschorz Palacos chirurg. 41:511.

Graham NB (1978) Polymeric inserts and implants for the controlled release of drugs. Br Polymer J 10:260–266.

Hernigou P, Thiery JP, Benoit J et al (1987) Release of antimitotic drugs from acrylic cement and plaster. Eur Surg Res 19(suppl 1):25.

Hernigou P, Thiery JP, Benoist M et al (1987) Etude experimentale sur l'osteosarcome d'une chimiotherapie locale diffusant a partir de ciment acrylique chirurgical et de platre. Rev Chir Orthop 73:517–525.

Hernigou P, Thiery JP, Benoit J et al (1989) Methotrexate diffusion from acrylic cement. Bone Joint Surg 71-B:804–811.

Hernigou P, Brun P, Thiery JP et al (1991) Antimitotic loaded acrylic cement. In: Langlais F (ed) Limb salvage. Springer Verlag, Berlin.

Hernigou Ph, Brun B, Autier A et al (1993) Osteosarcoma in adolescent and young adults. Kluwer Academic Publishers, Boston.

Hernigou Ph, Brun B, Autier A et al (1993) Diffusion of methotrexate from acrylic surgical cement. Cancer Treatment Res 62:231–235.

Hoff SH, Fitzgerald RH Jr, Kelly PJ (1981) The depot administration of penicillin G and gentamicin in acrylic bone cement. J Bone Joint Surg 63-A:798–804.

Janmin Li (1989) Experimental observations on acrylic bone cement containing antitumour drugs. Natl Med J China 69:143.

Klein B, Pals S, Masse R et al (1977) Studies of bone and soft-tissue tumours induced in rats with radioactive cerium chloride. Int J Cancer 10: 112–119.

Langendorff HU (1989) Cytostatic bone cement. In: Yamamuro T (ed) New developments for limb salvage in musculoskeletal tumours. Springer Verlag, Berlin.

Part 4

Radiotherapy

8 Radiotherapy in the Treatment of Bone Metastases

Th. Pignon, E. Cretel and P. Juin

8.1 Introduction

Bone is a common site of carcinoma metastases. Throughout the evolution of their disease, 25–50% of patients develop bone metastases. Approximately half of breast, prostate and lung cancers produce bone metastases, representing 75% of cases (Arcangeli et al, 1989; Price et al, 1986). Other cancers that may produce this secondary disease include colorectal, kidney, bladder and uterine cancer, and melanoma (Arcangeli et al, 1989). Median survival time for patients with bone metastases is 38–48 months (Perez et al, 1990; Toma et al, 1993), necessitating a safe and efficient treatment, which also gives a long-lasting effect.

External local radiotherapy remains the major treatment of bone metastasis, despite the fact that management by X-ray is not homogeneous. The main reasons for using radiation therapy are to relieve local bone pain, to prevent pathological fracture and vertebral collapse, and to promote healing in pathological fracture and relief of spinal cord compression. Systemic radiation therapy using beta-emitting radionucleotides is performed when pain becomes generalised, and causes less bone marrow toxicity than total or hemibody external irradiation.

Whatever method is employed, the role of radiotherapy is essentially palliative, to improve the patient's mobility, function and quality of life. However, there is still a considerable lack of agreement on optimal radiotherapy in each of the situations mentioned above (Bates et al, 1992).

8.2 External Radiotherapy

External radiotherapy can be delivered using local or wide-field irradiation. High-energy photons are now employed, whose energy will be adapted in relation to the depth of treatment.

8.2.1 Effect on Pain for Localised Bone Metastases

The pathogenesis of metastatic bone pain and its relief by radiotherapy are not completely understood. Reduction in tumour volume can explain relief of pain related to periosteal and nerve root compression, but cannot explain the rapid pain relief that can follow both local and extended radiotherapy. In addition, it is impossible to link onset of pain relief with tumour histology (Jensen and Roesdahl, 1976). Other mechanisms must be involved, which may act on cells that secrete the chemical mediators of the pain response, such as prostaglandins (Bates, 1992; Hoskin et al, 1992; Price et al, 1986).

As response does not differ according to histological type, all bone metastases can be managed with radiation therapy, although some data indicate more pain relief in breast and prostate cancer than in non-small-cell lung cancer carcinoma or renal adenocarcinoma (Arcangeli et al, 1989). Results seem to depend on the location of the bone metastases. Bone disease in the pelvis and inferior limbs responds less often to radiotherapy compared with other sites (Tong et al, 1982; Arcangeli et al, 1989). The median duration of response is longer in patients with total pain control at the end of radiotherapy than in others (25 vs 4 months).

Many retrospective studies failed to correlate pain relief to total dose delivered, dose-fractionation or tumour histology (Allen et al, 1976; Gilbert et al, 1977; Jensen and Roesdahl, 1976). Thus, a wide variety of irradiation schemes were designed, with approximately 80% of success with pain related to localised bone metastases (Garmatis and Chu, 1978). Delivering a single fraction has been reported to be as effective as multiple fractionation in several retrospective studies (Hendrickson et al, 1976; Penn, 1976; Qasim, 1977). In contrast, conventional radiation therapy giving 40 Gy or more in five daily fractions of 2–3 Gy was found to give better results in a retrospective analysis (Arcangeli et al, 1989). Therefore, fractionation schedules remain controversial. In a UK survey conducted in 1989, clinical oncologists were asked how they would manage a woman with a solitary painful breast cancer metastasis in her lumbar spine. The 168 respondents recommended 40 different regimens, ranging from 8 to 36 Gy in one to 15 fractions (Priestman et al, 1989). Institutional policy and patterns of training were among the more important reasons for this diversity of practice.

More evidence could be drawn from prospective studies. However, discrepancies between results have left the debate largely open. Numerous prospective randomised studies have shown similar efficacy using short hypofractionated regimens compared with schemes with higher doses delivered over longer periods. Price et al (1986) compared 8 Gy in one fraction with 30 Gy in ten fractions and found equal pain control in terms of response rate, and beginning and duration of pain relief during a period of at least 3 months, whatever the metastatic location and histological type of tumour. More recently, the same author showed a better effect with retreatment using 8 Gy in one fraction when compared with 4 Gy in one fraction (Hoskin et al, 1992). Cole (1989) supported these data, reporting earlier pain relief with a single fraction of 8 Gy than after 24 Gy in six fractions. In addition, patients who did not respond to a single fraction did so when retreated. Another controlled trial demonstrated comparable efficacy using 20 Gy in two fractions and 8 days or 25 Gy in six fractions and 18 days (Madsen, 1983). In a study on bone metastases of breast cancer, results were identical in the two treatment groups: 30 Gy in ten fractions or 15 Gy in three fractions (Rasmusson et al, 1995). The same result was found when comparing a single dose of 10 Gy to 22.5 Gy in five fractions, without improving toxicity (Gaze et al, 1997).

Short fractionation schemes are more comfortable for patients in pain, and treatment is simpler and less costly. Results of trials must be interpreted with caution, however, as many conclusions have been limited by the use of unreliable measures of response. Pain relief is usually assessed only by the physician, without self-evaluation by the patient, leading to misinterpretation of results. This was illustrated in a study by the Radiation Therapy Oncology Group, which investigated a large number of patients. Using physician assessment of pain relief, it was suggested that there was no relationship between total dose/fraction number and pain relief (Tong et al, 1982). A reanalysis of the data using different endpoints, including the need for retreatment, analgesic requirements and a pain score, concluded the opposite: that protracted dose fractionation schedules produced more pain relief than did short courses (Blitzer, 1985). Self-assessment of pain by the patient is generally more accurate than physician evaluation, particularly if more than one physician is involved. Combined evaluation, with the patient and the physician using validated criteria, seems the most appropriate way to provide reliable results.

Although many issues in treating bone metastasis remain unanswered, it seems preferable to treat patients with a short life expectancy using a single dose or hypofractionation schedule. When long-term survival is expected, as in breast or prostate cancer, late complications of radiation therapy may occur, so conventional radiotherapy is more appropriate.

8.2.2 Management of Multiple Bone Metastases

In patients suffering from multiple bone metastases, it may be difficult to define a target for efficient local radiotherapy. In this situation, hemibody radiotherapy has significant effects within 48 h (Salazar et al, 1986). A single fractionation dose of 6–8 Gy is generally delivered to the part of the body where more painful bone lesions are located. In addition, it is possible to give a second hemibody treatment to the opposite half if pain recurs in this site after an initial hemibody treatment. A booster dose can also be delivered to a localised painful area if pain relief is not sufficient.

This radiotherapy schedule does not generally have any adverse effects. Nausea is the most frequent acute effect, which is controlled by prophylactic anti-emetic drugs and adequate hydration. No cases of late morbidity have yet been reported following a single fraction of up to 8 Gy.

8.2.3 Prevention and Management of Pathological Fractures

Only 10% of bone metastases develop into pathological fractures. They can occur without being preceded by pain. These lesions are seen in high-risk patients with lytic lesions in weight-bearing bones, with more than 50% cortical destruction or a lytic diameter greater than 2.5 cm. Irradiation of the bone is generally recommended after surgical prophylactic fixation. Good results have been obtained in a retrospective study with a total dose of 30 Gy in ten daily fractions (Cheng et al, 1980).

Surgical fixation of a fracture is required to increase pain control and promote a more rapid return of mobility. An expected life duration of less than 6 weeks is not an absolute contraindication to surgery, as it may be the only way to ameliorate quality of life. Many retrospective studies have underlined the role of postoperative radiotherapy in pain relief and tumour reduction, although doses greater than 30 Gy in ten fractions could inhibit osteoblastic activity and interfere with bone healing. In one study, however, patients treated with 40 Gy in 20 fractions had a longer prognosis than average. Thus, in spite of a theoretical adverse effect of radiotherapy on bone healing, it seems that irradiation may help pain relief and recalcification by controlling local tumours (Ford and Yarnold, 1983).

However, optimal indications as well as the dose and fractionation of prophylactic or postoperative radiotherapy have to be confirmed by prospective randomised trials.

8.2.4 Management of Spinal Cord Compression due to Bone Metastases

Spinal cord compression is usually seen in patients with advanced metastatic disease, although it can be an initial sign of disease in 8% of cases (Gilbert and Prosser, 1978).

Prevention of spinal cord compression by radiotherapy is possible. In the case of recent vertebral collapse, radiotherapy should be started without waiting for pain or neurological signs. The efficacy of radiotherapy depends on its prompt initiation.

Management of spinal cord compression involves surgery with postoperative radiotherapy or radiotherapy alone. Improvement in neurological status is inversely proportional to the degree of neurological injury before treatment. There have been no prospective trials comparing radiotherapy with surgery, but radiotherapy does not have the same immediate effect on compression as surgery, nor does it restore the stability of a vertebra with severe collapse.

Candidates for radiotherapy are patients with progressive development of symptoms, cauda equina lesions or several compression levels, without vertebral instability or major compression. Radiotherapy is also used for patients with contraindications to surgery. Conventional radiotherapy delivers 25–40 Gy in a daily fraction of 2 Gy. Experimental data have shown than higher doses by fraction are more effective than lower doses. Thus, radiotherapy often begins with a high dose per fraction of 3 or 4 Gy until 15–20 Gy is reached. After several days of rest, radiotherapy can be continued with conventional fractionation or hypofractionation (Bates, 1992). A single-fraction dose also has a similar benefit. Results depend on the neurological status of the patient at the beginning of treatment. In selected cases, radiotherapy alone is as effective as surgery plus radiotherapy, with an improvement in the condition of almost half of patients. Conversely, in patients with bladder dysfunction or paraplegia, radiotherapy cannot ameliorate neurological status.

Postoperative radiotherapy leads to better functional and analgesic results than radiotherapy alone. In addition, the probability of recurrence is decreased.

Overall, results of surgery and/or radiotherapy are disappointing. In a literature review, Findlay (1984) found that only 38% of 1816 treated patients remained able to walk, or recovered the ability to walk. The best results were obtained in patients still able to walk before treatment, with 48, 67 and 79% of patients remaining ambulatory after surgery alone, surgery plus radiotherapy or radiotherapy alone, respectively. However, we cannot conclude that radiotherapy is the treatment of choice for all cases, as the best cases were probably selected for radiotherapy. When the tumour has a high radiosensitivity (multiple myeloma, lymphoproliferative tumours or germinal tumours), radiotherapy alone is efficient in more than 85% of cases (Janjan, 1996).

8.3 Systemic Radiotherapy

Systemic radiotherapy with radioactive isotope is an alternative approach to managing patients with multiple painful bone metastases.

Phosphorus-32 and strontium-89 are the radionucleotides most often used. The former has been demonstrated to be efficient in 50–70% of patients with severe hematotoxicity in 30% of cases. Strontium-89 is as effective as phosphorus but with less toxicity, having an asymptomatic decreasing rate of platelets and leukocytes in 30% of cases. Stontium-89 follows the pathways of calcium but, in contrast to phosphorus-32, it is not incorporated in bone marrow or leukocytes. It is preferentially retained in high-turnover sites, with a retention in metastatic sites of more than 90 days. Its biological half-life is 14 days in healthy people. Its potential toxicity is greater when the marrow has already undergone malignant infiltration. Contraindications include patients with inadequate levels of platelets and leukocytes in the peripheral circulation.

Reports using a dose of 40 μCi/kg gave an overall response of 79% in prostate cancer and 83% in breast cancer (Holmes, 1993), onset of pain relief beginning between 10 and 20 days after treatment (Laing et al, 1991). Increasing doses of strontium-89 have demonstrated no dose-response relationship and a dose range of 40–60 μCi/kg appears optimum for therapy.

In a prospective randomised trial, strontium-89 was as effective as local radiotherapy for relief of bone pain in prostate cancer and superior to conventional radiotherapy in delaying the progression of pain to new sites (Quilty et al, 1994). This result was consistent with another controlled study, which demonstrated that addition of strontium-89 to local radiotherapy delayed the progression of new sites of pain, and reduced the need for additional radiotherapy (Porter et al, 1993).

8.4 Summary

External local radiotherapy remains the major treatment of bone metastasis. Radiation therapy is usually performed to relieve local bone pain, to prevent pathological fracture and vertebral collapse, and to promote healing in pathological fracture and relief of spinal cord compression.

Systemic radiation therapy using beta-emitting radionucleotides is used in patients with generalised pain, giving less bone marrow toxicity than hemibody external irradiation. External radiotherapy with high-energy photons can be delivered for all bone metastases, as there is no difference of response according to histological type. Results seem to depend on the location of the bone metastases. Pelvic and inferior limb bone disease responds less often to radiotherapy than other sites.

Retrospective studies have failed to correlate pain relief with total dose delivered or dose-fractionation. Thus, a wide variety of irradiation schemes have been designed, with approximately 80% of success with pain related to localised bone metastases. Delivering a single fraction has been reported to be as effective as multiple fractionation in several retrospective studies. In contrast, conventional radiation therapy (five daily fractions of 2–3 Gy) was found to give better results in a retrospective analysis. Well-designed prospective studies are scarce, with generally unreliable results concerning the best radiotherapy scheme. However, it seems preferable to treat patients with a short life expectancy using a single dose or hypofractionation schedule. When long-term survival is expected, late complications of radiation therapy may occur, so a conventional radiotherapy schedule is more appropriate.

In spite of a theoretical adverse effect of radiotherapy on bone healing after surgical prophylactic fixation, irradiation may help pain relief and recalcification by controlling local tumours. Successful management of spinal cord compression by radiotherapy alone in certain selected patients gave good results in 85% of cases. In addition, systemic radiotherapy should be delivered postoperatively to decrease the probability of recurrence.

References

Allen KL, Jonhson TW, Hibbs GC (1976) Effective bone palliation as related to various treatment regimens. Cancer 37:984–987.

Arcangeli G, Micheli A, Arcangeli G et al (1989) The responsiveness of bone metastases to radiotherapy: the effect of site, histology and radiation dose on pain relief. Radiother Oncol 14:95–101.

Bates T (1992) A review of local radiotherapy in the treatment of bone metastases and cord compression. Int J Radiation Oncol Biol Phys 23:217–221.

Bates T, Yarnold JR, Blitzer P et al (1992) Bone metastasis consensus statement. Int J Radiation Oncol Biol Phys 23:215–216.

Blitzer PH (1985) Reanalysis of the RTOG study of the palliation of symptomatic osseous metastasis. Cancer 55:1468–1472.

Cheng DS, Seitz CB, Eyre HJ (1980) Non operative management of femoral, numeral and acetabular metastases in patients with breast carcinoma. Cancer 45:1533–1537.

Cole DJ (1989) A randomised trial of a single treatment versus conventional fractionation in the palliative radiotherapy of painful bone metastases. Clin Oncol 1:59–62.

Findlay GFG (1984). Adverse effects of the management of spinal cord compression. J Neurol Neurosurg Psychol 47:761–768.

Ford HT, Yarnold JR (1983) Radiation therapy, pain relief and recalcification. In: Stoll BA, Parbhoo S (eds) Bone metastases: monitoring and treatment. Raven Press, New York, pp 343–354.

Garmatis CJ, Chu FCH (1978) The effectiveness of radiation therapy in the treatment of bone metastases from breast cancer. Radiology 126:235–237.

Gaze MN, Kelly CG, Ker GR et al (1997) Pain relief and quality of life following radiotherapy for bone metastases: a randomised trial of two fractionation schedules. Radiother Oncol 45:109–116.

Gilbert HA, Kagan AR, Nussbaum H et al (1977) Evaluation of radiation therapy for bone metastases: pain relief and quality of life. Am J Roentgenol 129:1095–1096.

Gilbert RW, Kim JH, Prosser JB (1978) Epidural spinal cord compression from metastatic tumour: diagnosis and treatment. Ann Neurol 3:40–51.

Hendrickson FR, Shehata WM, Kirshner AB (1976) Radiation therapy for osseous metastasis. Int J Radiation Oncol Biol Phys 1:275–278.

Holmes RA (1993) Radiopharmaceuticals in clinical trials. Semin Oncol 20:22–26(suppl 2).

Hoskin PJ, Price P, Easton D et al (1992) A prospective randomised trial of 4 Gy or 8 Gy single doses in the treatment of metastatic bone pain. Radiother Oncol 23:74–78.

Janjan NA (1996). Radiotherapeutic management of spinal metastases. J Pain Symptom Management 11:47–56.

Jensen NH, Roesdahl K (1976). Single dose irradiation of bone metastasis. Acta Radiol Ther Phys Biol 15:337–339.

Laing AH, Ackery DM, Bayly RJ (1991) Strontium-89 chloride for pain palliation in prostatic skeletal malignancy. Br J Radiol 64:816–822.

Madsen EL (1983) Painful bone metastasis: efficacy of radiotherapy assessed by the patients: a randomised trial comparing 4 Gy x 6 versus 10 Gy x 2. Int J Radiation Oncol Biol Phys 9:1775–1779.

Penn CRH (1976) Single dose and fractionated palliative irradiation for osseous metastases. Clin Radiol 27:405–408.

Perez JE, Machiavelli M, Leone BA et al (1990) Bone-only versus visceral-only metastatic pattern in breast cancer: analysis of 150 patients. A GOCS study. Am J Clin Oncol 13:294–298.

Porter AT, McEwan AJB, Powe JE et al (1993) Results of a randomised phase III trial to evaluate the efficacy of strontium-89 adjuvant to local field external beam irradiation in the management of endocrine resistant metastatic prostate cancer. Int J Radiation Oncol Biol Phys 25:805–813.

Price P, Hoskin PJ, Easton D et al (1986) Prospective randomised trial of single and multifraction radiotherapy schedules in the treatment of painful bony metastases. Radiother Oncol 6:247–255.

Priestman T, Bullimore J, Godden T et al (1989) The Royal College of Radiologists' fractionation survey. Clin Oncol 1:39–46.

Qasim MM (1977). Single dose palliative irradiation for bone metastasis. Stralhentherapie 153:531–532.
Quilty PM, Kirk D, Dearnaley DP et al (1994) A comparison of the palliative effects of strontium-89 and external beam radiotherapy in metastatic prostate cancer. Radiother Oncol 31:33–40.
Rasmusson B, Vejborg I, Jensen AB et al (1995) Irradiation of bone metastases in breast cancer patients: a randomised study with 1 year follow-up. Radiother Oncol 34:179–184.
Salazar OM, Rubin P, Hendrickson FR et al (1986) Single-dose half-body irradiation for palliation of multiple bone metastases from solid tumours. Cancer 58:29–36.
Toma S, Venturino A, Sogno G et al (1993) Metastatic bone tumours. Non surgical treatment. Outcome and survival. Clin Orthopaed 295:246–251.
Tong D, Gillick L, Hendrickson FR (1982) The palliation of symptomatic osseous metastases. Cancer 50:893–899.

9 Radiosurgical Treatment of Bone Metastasis of the Limbs

Th. Pignon, P. Juin, Y. Glard and D.G. Poitout

9.1 Introduction

Bone metastases occur less frequently in the limbs than in the spine and pelvis. Metastases of the limbs are mainly found in the femur and humerus. The primary tumours from which they derive are: breast (30%), prostate (16%), lung (12%), kidney (10%), digestive system (6%) and thyroid (3%). In about 20% of cases, the origin of the primary tumour remains unknown. Bone metastases cause major discomfort because of the disability associated with fractures and/or pain. Survival should be assessed according to both disease progression and performance status, using the Karnofski score. Patients with a short survival time (2 weeks) require palliative treatment.

In most cases, treatment of bone metastasis is necessary. Surgery is required for osteolytic metastasis with a fracture or a threat of fracture because, although radiosurgical treatment may lead to recalcification, it is a long process. There is no need to perform an extensive and mutilating excision with non-pathological limits because treatment is in conjunction with radiosurgical treatment and eventual recovery is unlikely. Surgery may be necessary in patients with a single bone metastasis from kidney cancer because of the chance of a long survival and the poor radiosensitivity of the metastasis.

Radiosurgical treatment is very efficient in metastases of breast, prostate and thyroid cancers, leading to a decrease in pain in 80% of cases. It is also efficient in myeloma, which, although not a proper metastasis, causes similar problems.

Radiosurgical treatment is less efficient in cancers of the lung, digestive and urinary systems. Treatment is started as soon as the wound has healed, taking the whole bone as the irradiation volume and in some cases even overdosing the metastasis zone.

Although the presence of metallic prostheses, plates or screws affects the interaction of photons and material, we do not take this into account because of the very short distance covered by secondary electrons. Many surveys have shown that radiosurgical treatment concentrated over a short period of time is as efficient as identical doses of treatment spread over a longer time. We therefore use short courses.

We usually use one 30 Gy dose delivered in ten sessions or a 20 Gy dose delivered in five sessions. Single 8 Gy doses are used only as palliative treatment. Such treatment does not compromise any other later radioactive treatment, such as half-body treatment with phosphorus-32, Samarium or radioactive iodine.

The purpose of radiosurgical treatment is to provide efficient pain relief and to restore mobility in patients with at least a 10-month life expectation, making it easier to provide basic treatment for the illness. Although the average survival time is less for those with lung cancer, it is more for those with breast, kidney or thyroid cancers.

9.2 Patients

From 1986 to 1999, 831 cases of bone metastasis were selected, 127 of which had been treated for a metastasis in the long bone of the limb. Patients with scattered bone metastases (including limb metastases) were included only when they had been specifically treated. The femur was affected in more than 50% of cases (67/127); the humerus was the next most common site (26/127), then multiple bone metastases of the limbs (24/127), and finally the radius or tibia. The most common sites of primary tumour were the breast (52), lung (24) and prostate (22).

Only 15% of the patients did not feel any pain. Fractures were found in 8% of cases (12/127). Bone metastases of the limbs were associated with other bone metastases in 50% of cases and with visceral metastases in 25% of cases (32/127).

The average age of the group surveyed was 62.3 years (38–86 years). The average age of patients with prostate cancer was slightly higher (68.1 years), but this was not statistically significant. The average time between diagnosis of the primary tumour and diagnosis of the metastasis was 22 months (0–132 months).

The bone metastasis was known from the beginning in 41/127 cases. In 60/127 cases, radiosurgical treatment was performed, and 18/127 had surgery alone. Patients undergoing local treatment (breast and prostate) without any fracture received efficient general analgesics.

9.3 Methods

In more than 50% of cases, radiosurgical treatment delivered 30 Gy in ten sessions over 12 days. Telecobalt photons or more powerful photons delivered by a linear accelerator (15–18 MeV) were selected according to the thickness of the targeted bone.

The dose was calculated at half thickness on the basis of the field that first covered the whole long bone; it was then reduced to the metastatic volume when two-thirds of the dose had been delivered. Differences in thickness between the centre and the ends of the bone were taken into account using three computed tomography scan sections. The distal part of the femur received a 10% overdose, which was compensated for by excluding this zone during the last session. Each patient had a personal frame used to reduce irradiation on soft tissues. The frame setting could easily be modified from simulation shots.

The 28 other patients received various protocols (mainly 20 Gy in five sessions), particularly patients with lung cancer who were not in good health. In the eight cases receiving postoperative radiosurgical treatment, the dose was 30 Gy in seven sessions.

9.4 Results

No complications of radiosurgical treatment were observed. In 12 cases, radiosurgical treatment did not prevent a fracture, which was then treated surgically. Surgery was not complicated by the previous radiosurgical treatment.

Although it is difficult to analyse pain relief retrospectively, results of radiosurgical treatment were excellent in 22% of cases (28/127), good in 56% (71/127), poor in 16.5% (21/127) and bad in 5.5% (7/127). Results were scored as excellent when the pain relief was total, and good when the improvement was more than 75%, as assessed from the patient's statement and from the reduction in consumption of pain killer. In spite of the unrefined method of analysis, 78% of good or excellent results agrees with the published surveys.

9.5 Discussion

Except in special cases, single bone metastasis of a breast or thyroid primary tumour is compatible with a long survival. The diagnosis of bone metastasis means eventual death from this cause. Survival is greatly shortened in patients with lung cancer compared with prostate cancer.

The aim of local radiosurgical treatment treatment is not to eradicate the tumour, but to:

- Relieve pain, which is the first symptom
- Prevent or treat a fracture
- Maintain the patient's autonomy
- Improve the comfort and quality of life of the patient, making it easier to continue systemic treatment if necessary.

Radiosurgical treatment appears to be a very good analgesic treatment in about 78% of cases (the results are not so good in the case of primary tumours of the lung or digestive system).

In spite of real progress in the study of primary tumours and the pathophysiology of bone metastasis, the way in which radiosurgical treatment works remains poorly understood. Reduction in the tumour mass is likely to reduce compression on the periosteum or nerves. It is likely that the rapid action of radiosurgical treatment is a result of chemical mediators such as prostaglandin, particularly on a wide field, as in half-body irradiation.

Threat of a fracture is estimated to occur in 70% of cases, when more than half the cortex is destroyed. According to Cheng et al (1980), a 30 Gy dose of radiosurgical treatment would prevent this. However, Cheng's study looked only at bone metastasis of primary tumours in the breast. Erosion of the cortex and lytic characteristics of the bone metastasis seem to be good criteria for surgery, particularly for stressed bones such as the femur. Postoperative radiosurgical treatment should be performed systematically, provided the patient's health condition is good enough and the survival expectation is at least 3 months.

Until recently, a dose of 30 Gy in ten sessions was the most common protocol. Tong et al (1982), in a study for the Radiation Therapy Oncology Group, demonstrated that a single 8 Gy dose had the same results. On the other hand, Blitzer (1985), in a study of multiple and single metastases, came to a different conclusion. Arcangeli et al (1989) estimated that the best results are obtained by a split dose of 40 Gy or more. Price et al (1986) and Cole (1989) stated the benefit of a single 8 Gy dose, but not a 4 Gy dose.

Except in the case of an obvious threat of fracture, we deliver a single 8 Gy dose because this reduces the length of treatment and improves the patient's comfort. Moreover, if the treatment is not sufficient, it can be repeated. This treatment does not prevent half-body radiosurgical treatment if the bone metastases are multiple.

On the whole, pain relief is excellent. From 6 to 7 Gy doses are delivered on the upper body, and 7–8 Gy on the lower body, in a single session or two sessions separated by 2–4 weeks. Partial pain relief is achieved in 55–100% of cases and total relief in 5–50% of cases. The pain relief occurs after 1–14 days.

Side-effects such as nausea, vomiting, diarrhoea and sometimes medullar or lung toxicity may occur. These complications are found in 2–8% of cases after irradiation of the whole body and in 4–32% of cases after irradiation of the upper body.

9.6 Conclusion

Treatment of bone metastasis with radiosurgical treatment reduces pain and maintains mobility in patients with an average life expectancy of 10 months. Survival is lower in patients with lung cancer but higher in those with breast, kidney or thyroid cancer. As well as increasing the patient's comfort, radiosurgical treatment allows basic treatment of the illness to be continued.

References

Arcangeli G, Micheli A, Arcangeli G et al (1989) The responsiveness of bone metastases to radiotherapy: the effect of site, histology and radiation dose on pain relief. Radiother Oncol 14:95–101.

Blitzer PH (1985) Reanalysis of the RTOG study of the palliation of symptomatic osseous metastases. Cancer 55: 1468–1472.

Cheng DS, Seitz CB, Eyre HJ (1980) Nonoperative management of femoral, humeral, and acetabular metastases in patients with breast carcinoma. Cancer 45:1533–1537.

Cole DJ (1989) A randomized trial of single treatment versus conventional fractionation in the palliative radiotherapy of painful bone metastases. Clin Oncol 1:59–62.

Nielsen OS, Munro AJ, Tannock IF (1991) Bone metastases: pathophysiology and management policy. J Clin Oncol 9(3):509–524.

Price P, Hoskin PJ, Austin A et al (1986). Prospective randomized trial of single and multifraction radiotherapy schedules in the treatment of painful bone metastases. Radiother Oncol 6:247–255.

Tong D, Gillick L, Ilendrickson FR (1982) The palliation of symptomatic osseous metastases. Final results of the study by the Radiation Therapy Oncology Group. Cancer 50:893–899.

Further Reading

Bates T (1989) Radiotherapy for bone metastases. Clin Oncol 1:57–58.

Berrettoni BA, Carter JR (1986) Mechanisms of cancer metastases. J Bone Joint Surg 68:308–312.

Carter RL (1985) Patterns and mechanisms of localized bone by tumours: studies with squamous carcinomas of the head and neck. Crit Rev Clin Lab Sci 22:275–315.

Carter RL (1985) Patterns and mechanisms of bone metastases. J Royal Soc Med 78:2–6(suppl 9).
Fidler IJ, Radinsky R (1990) Genetic control of cancer metastases. J Natl Cancer Inst 82:166–168.
Hoskin PJ (1988) Scientific and clinical aspects of radiotherapy in the relief of bone pain. Cancer Surv 7:69–86.
Liotta LA, Steller Stevenson WG (1989) Principles of molecular cell biology of cancer; cancer metastases. In: De Vita VT, Hellman S, Rosenberg SA (eds) Cancer: principles and practice of oncology. JB Lippincott, Philadelphia, pp 98–115.
Lote K, Walloc A, Bjersand A (1986) Bone metastasis. Prognosis, diagnosis and treatment. Acta Radiol Oncol 25:227–232.
Malawel MM, Delaney TF (1989) Treatment of mestastasis cancer to bone. In: De Vita VT, Hellman S, Rosenberg SA (eds) Cancer: principles and practice of oncology. JB Lippincott, Philadelphia, pp 2298– 2317.
Mauch PM, Drew MA (1985) Treatment of metastatic cancer to bone. In: De Vita VT, Hellman S, Rosenberg SA (eds) Cancer: principles and practice of oncology. JB Lippincott, Philadelphia, pp 2132–2141.
Paterson AHG (1987) Bone metastasis in breast cancer, prostate cancer and myeloma. Bone 8:17–22(suppl 1).
Price P, Hoskin PJ, Easton D et al (1988) Low dose single fraction radiotherapy in the treatment of metastatic bone pain: a pilot study. Radiother Oncol 12:297–300.
Salazar OM, Rubin P, Hendrickson FR et al (1986) Single dose half-body irradiation for the palliation of multiple bone metastases from solid tumours. Int J Radiation Oncol Biol Phys 7:773–781.
Wagnor G (1984) Frequency of pain in patients with cancer. Recent Results Cancer Res 89:64–71.

Part 5

Surgical Treatment

10 Surgery for Bone Metastasis of the Limbs

D.G. Poitout, P. Tropiano, B. Clouet D'Orval, B. Ripoll and Y. Glard

10.1 Introduction

Unfortunately, the occurrence of a metastasis during the evolution of cancer means a bad prognosis. It is evidence of spreading of the pathology and in the end the victory of cancer over the organism.

However, present medical therapy (hormonal therapy, chemotherapy, radiotherapy) has increased patients' survival, making surgery for metastasis increasingly important.

Surgery for bone metastasis is palliative, with the following aims:

- Suppression of the pain associated with the metastasis
- Prevention of pathological fractures
- Stabilisation of the bone using osteosynthesis or a prosthesis
- Conservation of function, allowing rapid rehabilitation, continuation of medical treatment and an early return home.

The frequency of bone metastases is difficult to assess and usually underestimated. Bone metastases are more frequent than primary bone tumours. They are mainly caused by epithelial cancers, such as breast, prostate, lung, kidney and thyroid cancers. Nevertheless, any cancer can trigger bone metastases. They are most likely to be found in the spine and the femur, but any bone can be affected. Multifocal metastases are common, so a full bone check-up must be carried out. Although the overall prognosis is poor, mobility is threatened, so surgical treatment should be encouraged.

Surgery for bone metastases is palliative, because it does not lengthen the survival period, but it is also restorative, because the bone retrieves its original functional and morphological qualities.

Three clinical situations can lead to metastasis treatment:

- The primary cancer is known and under scrutiny. A routine scintigraphy or radiography may reveal a metastasis, usually an osteolytic one
- Investigation of pain or a fracture may reveal a metastasis in a patient who has already been diagnosed with cancer
- The metastasis may be prevalent, revealed after radiography to investigate localised pain, tumefaction or fracture.

The metastasis may reveal the site of the primary cancer. Bone biopsy is useful because the metastasis and the primary tumour are quite similar histologically.

10.2 Clinical Bases

From 1981 to 1999, we conducted a survey of 87 patients who had received preventive surgery for bone metastases of the limbs. The metastases had classical aetiologies (breast, kidney, lung, thyroid and prostate), but digestive cancers were also found in more than 10% of cases.

The metastases were mainly on the proximal extremities of the femur or the humerus. The material used depended on whether they were on the diaphysis or the epiphysis. Osteosynthesis may be preventive, or used for treatment of spontaneous fractures, and must provide stability. It must last for the rest of the patient's life, and surgical cement is often added to the osteosynthesis material.

10.2.1 The Femur

Several procedures are offered for treatment of metastases affecting the diaphysis.

Insertion of a nail, either locked or not, can avoid a surgical approach at the site of the metastasis, which may be haemorrhagic (such as metastasis from the kidney). It may be necessary to hold the lytic zone in place with dental forceps in order to remove the metastasis. This will avoid movement during the nailing process (particularly as a large nail and cement are used together).

A screwed plate or AO-95° plate allows the metastatic zone to be resected or filled with cement. The process consists of setting the plate and screwing the ends, then injecting fluid cement in both the proximal and distal segments after opening the bone cortex. Finally, during the plastic phase of polymerisation, the screwing is completed.

Treatment of metastases affecting the metaphysis involves use of AO-95° plates with cement or massive reconstruction prostheses.

10.2.2 The Humerus

Plates with cement or massive prostheses are used. Because a shorter upper limb is less disabling than a shorter lower limb, resection of the tumour is usually performed.

Patients should not be refused rehabilitation surgery, even if their prognosis is poor. Although treatment is only palliative, it can offer considerable relief during the remainder of the patient's life.

10.3 Principles of Palliative Surgery for Bone Metastasis

The treatment goals of palliative surgery are to:

- Relieve pain associated with metastasis
- Avoid a pathological fracture. If more than one-third of the cortex is damaged, there is a major risk of fracture. Irradiation of metastases may initially increase osteolysis
- Conserve or restore bone continuity, using osteosynthesis or a prosthesis

- Offer the best possible conservation of function
- Obtain immediate results with massive articular prostheses, allowing rapid return of mobility without waiting for bone consolidation
- Allow continuation of anticancer treatment, thus suppressing the effects of the metastasis.

Questions often asked about palliative surgery include:

- Do the patient's survival hopes make surgery worthwhile?
- Is focal surgery of bone metastasis harmless?
- Can bone consolidation be expected?
- Is excision of the metastatic tumour necessary?
- Does palliative surgery allow complementary radiotherapy?

The survival of patients with bone metastasis from breast cancer is only 22 months on average. Although survival is unpredictable, palliative surgery will at least provide pain relief.

The average survival period is the same with both orthopaedic and surgical treatment. According to the statistics, surgical trauma does not cause any local or general worsening of the condition.

Metastatic fractures consolidate in only 5–20% of cases after radiotherapy or hormone therapy, so consolidation cannot be expected after palliative surgery. The osteosynthesis has to be stable and definitive, taking into account osteolysis and the poor quality of the bone.

Total excision of the tumour can stop bleeding in some haemorrhagic metastatic tumours that cannot be controlled by preoperative arterial embolisation. Moreover, when there is only one metastasis, reduction in tumour volume can reinforce the medical treatment. Carcinological resection of bone metastasis may be considered in young patients whose health is otherwise good.

Nowadays, materials used for osteosynthesis or prostheses are compatible with radiotherapy. Radiotherapy must start as soon as a skin scar has formed. It can slow down the local progression of metastasis and may lead to recalcification of the affected bone, and even to consolidation of a pathological fracture. Doses of 8–40 Gy are used, according to the volume and the site of the metastasis.

10.4 Methods

Until the 1960s, orthopaedic treatment was the only method used to treat bone metastases. Bedridden patients often died of complications resulting from immobility. With the use of acrylic cements, prostheses allowed the treatment of lesions near the joints. Centro-medullar nails were first used successfully on the diaphysis. To obtain a stable osteosynthesis, the tumour cavity and the diaphysis can be filled with cement, through which the nail is set and the plate screwed on each side of the tumour.

On the lower limbs, metastases mainly affect the femur, particularly the upper extremity. For palliative osteosynthesis, the material needs to be deeply rooted in the proximal fragment. It is limited to the area below and around the trochanter. An AO plate, or DHS or THS screwed plate is used, and the tumour cavity is filled with cement. If the patient's general health is poor, use of Ender's nails may be necessary, allowing at least mobilisation and nursing, at best weight-bearing on the limb. In healthier patients, a cemented prosthesis may be necessary if early weight-bearing is required. Standard reconstruction prostheses allow a large resection of the upper extremity of the femur. A long shaft prosthesis should be used in cases of tiered metastases.

If the acetabulum is affected, the acetabulum-like part of the prosthesis will be held by a ring screwed in the healthy bone around and above the acetabulum.

Femoral metastases on the diaphysis are treated using long screwed plates and osteosynthesis with cement, or a centro-medullar nail with or without cement.

For humeral metastases, particularly those on the upper metaphysis, treatment is usually with a cemented plate, but a prosthesis may be used for the upper extremity of the humerus. However, the functional results of such a prosthesis are quite disappointing.

Other areas of the limbs are less frequently affected. Metastasis of the limb tips can lead to distal amputation if there is ulceration, although this is not recommended as it does not help treatment.

10.5 Discussion

Various surgical treatments are available for bone metastases. Although patients are terminally ill, surgery for multiple bone metastases may be offered to those in fairly good health, and the patient will benefit from the analgesic effect of osteosynthesis.

To avoid spontaneous fracture, preventive osteosynthesis should be performed in a patient with pain or significant cortical destruction, particularly on the lower limbs.

The patient will require brief mobility re-training in a specialised centre, but it is important for him to return home as quickly as possible, even if the re-education is not complete.

10.6 Conclusion

Discovery of a primary tumour and its metastasis to bones and viscera are not reasons for refusing the patient the benefit of rehabilitation surgery. Even if the surgery is palliative, it can offer the patient worthwhile relief during his survival.

The frequency of metastasis is rising because the survival of patients with spreading cancer has increased as a result of improvements in medical treatments.

Basic procedures for the surgery of limbs affected by bone metastases are palliative osteosynthesis and massive prostheses, followed by radiotherapy. The mechanical qualities of the materials used have been improved to lengthen their life duration. New procedures are offered for particular areas (acetabulum, upper extremity of the humerus, spine).

When there is only one bone metastasis from a primary tumour that is being controlled medically, carcinological surgery will be beneficial.

11 Surgical Treatment of Vertebral Metastases

R. Louis, Ch. Louis, R. Aswad and P. Tropiano

Before the 1970s, the appearance of a vertebral metastasis meant rapid deterioration and death for the patient; the only treatment was prescription of major analgesic drugs. Patients suffered dramatic and precocious paralyses secondary to radiculo-spinal cord compression. The introduction of spinal internal fixation, in the 1970s, has allowed stabilisation of the metastatic spine, with unexpected disappearance of pain. The use of osteosynthesis enables paralysed patients to recuperate. If the surgical procedure is carried out before the nervous compression has begun, osteosynthesis prevents the development of paralysis. Patients have been able to continue their activities and remain comfortable for the remainder of their lives.

Since the 1980s, progress in chemotherapy, hormone therapy and cobalt radiotherapy, in association with surgery, has considerably lengthened the life expectancy of patients with a metastatic spine. Management of the metastatic spine, like that of bony primitive tumours, has necessarily become multidisciplinary.

Metastasis of the spine is a malignant process developing in one or several vertebrae, originating from the primitive tumour located elsewhere. The nature of the primitive tumour is breast cancer in 30% of cases, unknown cancer in 16%, lung cancer in 13%, kidney cancer in 12%, prostate cancer in 7%, gastrointestinal cancer in 7%, thyroid cancer in 5% and various other cancers in 9% (Nazarian et al, 1997). Brihaye et al (1988) give a lower percentage of metastases originating from breast cancer (16.5% from breast cancer and 12.5% from unknown primitive lesions). Thirty-six per cent of patients die of spinal metastasis, with only 52% of lesions visible on simple radiographs and 26% visible histologically but not radiologically (Wong et al, 1990).

The distribution of metastases in the spine is proportional to the height of each vertebral segment: cervical 24%, thoracic 48%, lumbar 26%, sacral 2% (Nazarian et al, 1997). Metastatic disease of the spine most frequently affects patients aged 50–60 years. The vertebral pathway of the metastases seems to be essentially venous through the intraspinal venous plexus (Batson, 1940). The vertebral venous system normally drains 5–10% of the whole body venous system (Louis, 1983). Because of its significant vascularisation, the bone marrow provides a propitious environment for the development of the cancerous emboli. The vertebral bodies are therefore 20 times more receptive to metastases than the posterior elements. Only 3–4% of metastases are localised in the epidural space (Brihaye et al, 1988).

The metastases create a cancellous bony resorption secondary to remodelling osteoclastic activity, which may also be mediated by prostaglandin secretion. The result is vertebral weakening under the axial constraints of the spine, progressing first to microscopical fractures of the trabeculae, followed by vertebral collapse.

The vertebral pain is more often a result of the fracture than of the direct invasion of the tumour into the intrinsic nervous tract of the spine. Thus, the neurological lesion is frequently the result of anterior compression of the dura, the spinal cord or roots of the cauda equina caused by the rupture of the posterior wall of a collapsed vertebra. More rarely, the nervous lesion is the consequence of arterial disruption by tumour invasion with thromboses, especially when the whole epidural space is invaded by a primitive or secondary tumour. Paralytic lesions are more frequent at the thoracic level, where the epidural space is relatively narrow; vertebral body collapse is therefore more likely to occur in the thoracic kyphotic spine.

Treatment of spinal metastases has two components: local, to stabilize the spine, to reduce the pain and to prevent or restore neurological lesions; and general, to treat the disease, with a choice of chemotherapy, hormone therapy, cobalt therapy or immunotherapy.

11.1 Therapeutic Decision

The therapeutic decision will be made after a full investigation of the disease to determine the indications or contraindications to surgery and to specify the strategy for using the various treatments associated with surgery.

11.1.1 Investigations

The first signs of vertebral metastases are local pain along the spine in 97.4% of cases and nerve root pain in 56.5% of cases. Sensory motor deficits affect 45% of patients and sphincter dysfunction 21% (Nazarian et al, 1997). Visible radiographic signs on standard X-rays are delayed. Radiography may demonstrate one or two missing pedicles and vertebral collapse with an osteolytic lesion; sometimes sclerotic areas can be found. Bone scintigraphy is generally positive but non-specific and does not reveal the extent of the lesions. The most sensitive and specific investigation is magnetic resonance imaging with injection of gadolinium. This enables the limits of the metastasis to be defined and therefore its locoregional extension.

However, the best diagnostic tool is biopsy, which can be percutaneous or performed using an open approach. Some osteoporotic fractures with vertebral collapse in elderly patients can simulate a metastasis, but in this case the pedicles are not affected. In other cases, a latent infectious syndrome should be eliminated. However, the vertebral disc is not affected by malignant tumours, whereas it may be collapsed in infectious conditions. Percutaneous biopsy is carried out with either a small or a large needle, in the osteolytic area of the tumour if possible, with a positive average rate of 75%. Haemorrhage occurs in 0.7% of cases; this may be lethal or lead to neurological complications. Biopsy material should be sent to the laboratory routinely, not only for histological study but also for culture to rule out indolent infections. The aspirated blood should also be analysed. Open-approach biopsy is performed by a transpedicular posterior approach, using a curette, on the osteolytic zone, only in the thoracic and lumbar regions. For cervical lesions, an anterior approach is more adequate and safe, with minimal morbidity.

Laboratory tests, particularly a platelet count, are necessary before surgery is considered, to evaluate the haemostatic status of the patient. Furthermore, laboratory tests allow evaluation of the general impact of the cancerous disease on the patient, particularly by assessing the degree of anaemia. The dosage of tumour markers is useful. Liver ultrasound and thoracic radiography allow assessment of metastatic extensions to these structures. Finally, selective angiography localises the Adamkiewicz artery and allows preoperative embolisation of the tumour arteries, decreasing surgical bleeding before all extensive surgery, and especially surgery anterior to the thoracic and lumbar spine.

Numerous classifications have been proposed to describe the clinical presentation of patients to determine the therapeutic indications (De Wald et al, 1985; Tokuhashi et al, 1990). In reality, on final evaluation, one should know that the lesion is a metastasis, isolated or multiple, intra- or extracortical, with nervous compression or spinal cord ischaemia, especially in acute neurological lesions leading to complete paralysis. Progressive insidious evolution with upper motor neurone findings is a result of insidious compression. Furthermore, one should know if the spine is stable or not, whether the contiguous bone is normal or osteoporotic, whether there is some associated metastasis, and whether the patient has more or less than 6 months of life expectancy.

11.1.2 Surgical Indications and Contraindications

Surgery is contraindicated when life expectancy is likely to be less than 6 months as a result of deterioration of the patient or the presence of liver, lung or brain metastases. Sometimes, haemostatic dysfunction can temporarily contraindicate surgical treatment. Multiple metastases on an osteoporotic spine can also contraindicate surgical stabilisation because of the poor mechanical bone quality. External stabilization is indicated when surgical fixation is impossible. This can be done using a thoracolumbar plastic brace or a craniothoracic halo.

The best surgical indication is an isolated intracortical vertebral metastasis in a healthy patient. The surgical goal is then to remove the lesion completely in one or two steps, restoring and stabilizing the three pillars of the spine. Vertebroplasty can be proposed for an isolated intracortical lesion, if the posterior wall is not damaged. The presence of an extracortical lesion to one or more adjacent vertebral bodies, with or without insidious neurological compression, may indicate an anterior approach for tumourectomy and anterior decompression with reconstruction and internal fixation. A vertebral metastasis with incomplete neurological impairment and partial or complete osteolysis of the posterior structure can be treated by a posterior approach with reconstruction and stabilisation. Patients with acute complete paralysis are usually bad candidates for surgery because the surgical procedure has no effect on ischaemia, but may accelerate death. Only cases diagnosed early, before complete paralysis, can benefit from a posterior surgical decompression approach with stabilization.

11.1.3 Therapeutic Strategy

The place of adjuvant treatment in therapy can be determined only by a multidisciplinary consultation between the surgeon, the radiotherapist and the oncologist. Hormone therapy, particularly useful in cancer of the prostate and breast, can be administered, pre- and postoperatively, as soon as the lesion is diagnosed. Chemotherapy and immunotherapy expose the patient to thrombopenia, with a risk of bleeding, and to neutropenia, with bone marrow aplasia and a risk of infection. It will therefore be necessary to delay these therapies until 15 days after the operation. Surgical treatment for neurological lesions takes priority over adjuvant treatment. A low analgesic dose of radiotherapy (less than 20 Gy) can be used preoperatively. High curative doses of radiotherapy (40 Gy) should be reserved for the postoperative period, after wound healing. After intensive radiotherapy preceding a large double-approach surgical procedure, spinal cord ischaemia may appear postoperatively because the radiation may have caused an arteritis that, added to the effect of the surgical haemostasis, will decrease the spinal cord circulation, leading to irreversible paraplegia.

11.2 Surgical Techniques

There are three categories of surgical technique: vertebroplasty, limited surgery and extensive surgery or total vertebrectomy.

11.2.1 Vertebroplasty

The vertebroplasty method was developed by Deramond et al (1990). The process involves injecting cement (acrylic) into the body of a pathological vertebra, using a percutaneous needle. The technique is performed under direct digital radioscopy (in an angiography room) with a mobile radioscopy machine, allowing an anteroposterior and lateral view. An anterolateral approach is used for the cervical spine, with the patient in a decumbent position, directing the needle between the digestive tract and the vessels. The transpedicle and posterolateral approaches are possible for the lumbar and thoracic regions, with the patient in a procumbent position.

Progression of the cement into the vertebral body should be followed during the injection, to check that there is no leak likely to cause neurological compression. If cement leaks into the venous system of the vertebral body, the injection must be stopped and the needle removed, as this can lead to pulmonary embolism. A leak into the intervertebral disc has no serious consequences. Cement may leak into peri- or intraspinal soft tissue if the cortex of the vertebral body is ruptured or if the bone is fragile. Follow-up after vertebroplasty is simple and the patient can leave hospital on the third or fourth day. Some patients have inflammatory pain, which may be relieved by steroids or non-steroid anti-inflammatory drugs.

The vertebroplasty technique allows good stabilisation and analgesia of the diseased vertebra, but it is essential that the cortex has not collapsed. In isolated and intracortical metastases, surgery increases life expectancy to a greater extent than vertebroplasty. If surgery is contraindicated because preliminary high doses of radiotherapy have been given, vertebroplasty is the favoured method. For the cervical spine, vertebroplasty is less invasive than surgery and is therefore preferred. If the vertebra is fragile after decompression-fusion of the posterior wall, vertebroplasty will consolidate the anterior pillar.

11.2.2 Limited Surgery for Vertebral Metastases

Either the posterior or anterior approach, or sometimes both, is used. Angiography with embolisation is a good preoperative precaution.

11.2.2.1 Posterior Approach

Whatever the spinal level, this approach is almost always the same, with a median posterior incision. After radiographic tracking, one or two vertebrae are exposed above and below the injured level. It is often preferable to begin the laminectomy in a healthy zone away from the injured part, to ensure easy visualisation of the dura if there is epiduritis. Sometimes the laminectomy has to be extensive to one or two posterior pillars of the facets and the pars interarticularis to suppress the tumour site or to decompress one or several foramina. The epiduritis should be completely excised along the dura, avoiding spinal cord trauma, from the atlas to L2, using root retractors.

For haemostasis, we use electrocoagulation, a haemostatic pack and bony wax with moist hot gauze. Some operations are very haemorrhagic and anaesthesia causing arterial hypotension should be avoided because there is a risk of spinal cord ischaemia. Intraoperative transfusions compensate for blood loss. When the dura is sufficiently decompressed, the vertebrae are stabilised by internal fixation using plates, hook-rods or wire-rods, extending to one or two healthy vertebrae above and below the decompression (Fig. 11.1).

With the posterior approach, the use of methylmethacrylate cement to replace excised posterior pillars is not desirable because there is a significant risk of nerve compression. If the life expectancy of the patient is more than 6–12 months, we use autogenous cancellous iliac grafts, all along the posterior pillars and the internal hard material. Sometimes, when there are two different lesion levels posteriorly, we can perform the same operation for the two levels. The surgical wound is closed on a sucking drain. In malnourished patients or in those who have already undergone radiotherapy, sutures should be removed after the third week. For the upper cervical spine, stabilisation is ensured by occipito-cervical plating or by use of a temporary halo for a few months. For sacral metastases, we use a setting made with four crossing plates, two horizontal plates passing on the sacrum and screwed on the external iliac fossa after bending the plates, then two vertical plates, bolted to the horizontal ones and fixed to the pedicles of the last two lumbar vertebrae.

11.2.2.2 Anterior Approach

When metastatic lesions affect the vertebral bodies with or without anterior compression of the dura, particularly when there is a compression fracture, it is often more judicious and efficient to operate by an anterior approach to correct the deformity, to re-establish the solidity of the anterior pillar and to adapt an osteosynthesis. A transoral or lateropharyngeal approach may be used for the cervical spine. A classical anterolateral approach may be used for the lower cervical spine and the upper thoracic spine (T1–T2). A transpleural approach, in a dorsal

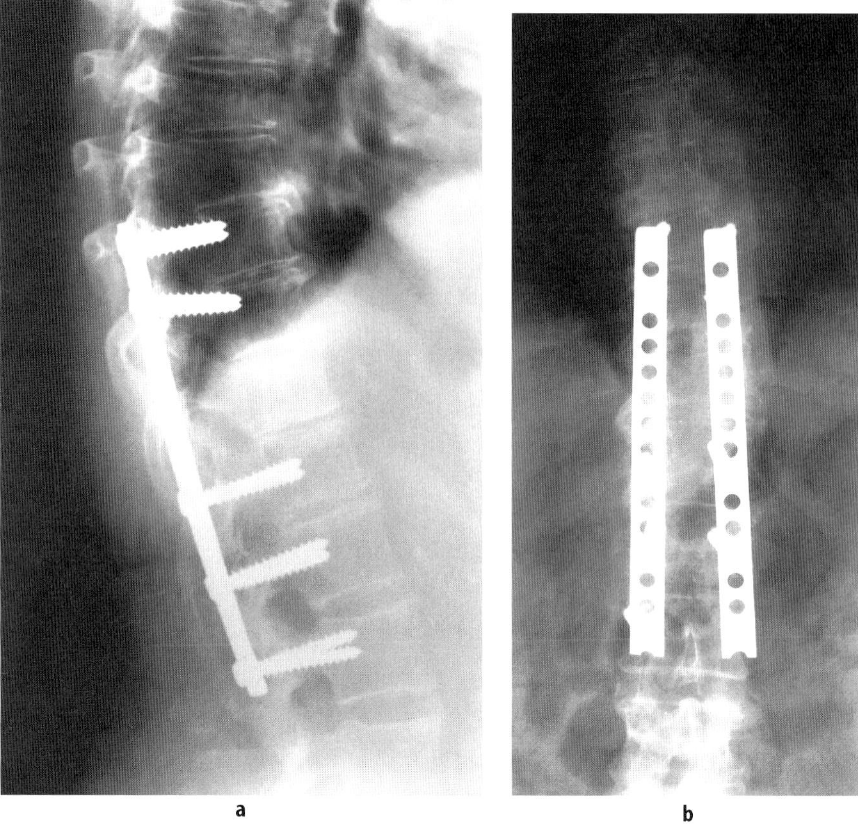

Figure 11.1 **a** Operative result of a T11 metastasis. Posterior decompression and internal fixation with a plate from L2 to T8. **b** Anteroposterior view. The patient survived, with mild pain, for 13 months after the surgery

or lateral decumbent position, may be used for the thoracic spine. The thoracolumbar junction, the lumbar spine and the lumbosacral junction may require a left thoraco-phreno-lombotomy, a left anterolateral approach and a sub- or transperitoneal approach respectively.

For operation on a patient with significant deformity of the spine, mild lordosing traction may be required, using a leather helmet or a halo for the head, shoes fixed to the operating table for the feet, and an angulated table or a bolster under the deformity. A dynamometer is used to prevent excessive traction (5–10 kg for the cervical spine and 15–20 kg for the thoracolumbar spine). The traction can be applied only if the posterior structures are still solid. To avoid altering the blood circulation in the spinal cord during operations on the thoracic and lumbar spine, haemostasis of segmental vessels on one side of the spine and at equal distances from the median line and the foramina is recommended, avoiding damage to the foramina, where the arteries cross. It is better not to perform an anterior approach if the patient has already undergone intensive radiotherapy. The injured vertebral bodies are excised with a curette as far as the opening of the vertebral canal. The curette, particularly the angulated type, may be manipulated from the deep to the superficial area, thus avoiding harm to the spinal cord.

During the excision, haemostasis should be ensured using Surgicel, moist and hot gauze and bony wax. The healthy vertebral endplates adjacent to the tumour are cleaned of fibrous tissue and cartilage, but their solid cortex is retained for the setting. If there is a spinal cord lesion, the posterior vertebral longitudinal ligament also has to be excised up to the anterior aspect of the dura. Two layers of Surgicel allow protection of the dura and ensure haemostasis of epidural veins. Reduction is generally obtained by application of the three forces of the lordosing vertebral traction, without needing other mechanical actions. Reconstruction of the great anterior pillar (vertebral bodies and discs) is usually done with methylmethacrylate cement, used to fill the excised zone. The fixation on each intact endplate that limits the excised area can be improved by a small anchoring hole. Placing Surgicel against the dura avoids heat transmission while the cement hardens. Internal stabilization is necessary, using either a screwed plate with two or three screws in each of the adjacent healthy vertebral bodies, or rods with hooks or screws (Fig. 11.2). Sometimes the loss of substance can be compensated by solid autogenous graft, such as a fibula, or by Harms' metallic cages, filled with autogenous cancellous grafts and supported on the extreme endplates. Substitutes proposed by various companies are not always reliable in the long term. After closing the wound with sucking drainage, the patient may require external support (brace or minerva plaster) for a few months.

For patients presenting with lesions in both the vertebral body and posterior structures, a double approach may be necessary.

11.2.3 Vertebrectomy

It is not possible to use vertebrectomy for monobloc excision of a vertebral tumour site, but it is a more satisfactory and sophisticated technique than vertebroplasty or limited surgery. Total vertebrectomy may be used to remove both the vertebral body and the the posterior structures of the lesion.

For the thoracic spine, total vertebrectomy is possible only by a posterior approach, following the technique of Roy-Camille et al (1985). This operation requires preoperative angiography because the radiculo-medullary arteries pass at the level of several foramina. We prefer the double-approach vertebrectomy, usually separated by a week. A double approach allows us to work in front of and behind the foramina without having to cut the vessels at their levels, respecting the anastomotic vessels after ligature and section of the metameric vessels (Fig. 11.3).

This technique is indicated only for healthy well-nourished patients, whose life expectancy is more than 6 months and who have lesions limited to the spine, particularly intracortical lesions. The first approach is the one that allows the best neurological decompression when there are associated signs of paralysis. For each approach, posterior and anterior, the posterior structures and the vertebral body respectively will be completely excised. The repair should be done at the level of each of the three pillars (Louis' theory) (Louis, 1983), the great pillar anteriorly and the two posterior pillars made by the succession of the pars interarticulares and facets (Fig. 11.4). For reconstruction of the pillars, we prefer to use autogenous fibular struts for the vertebral bodies in one or two struts according to the diameter of the vertebral body, and iliac grafts for the posterior pillars. The internal fixation will also have to be triple for the pillars. We prefer lateral screwed

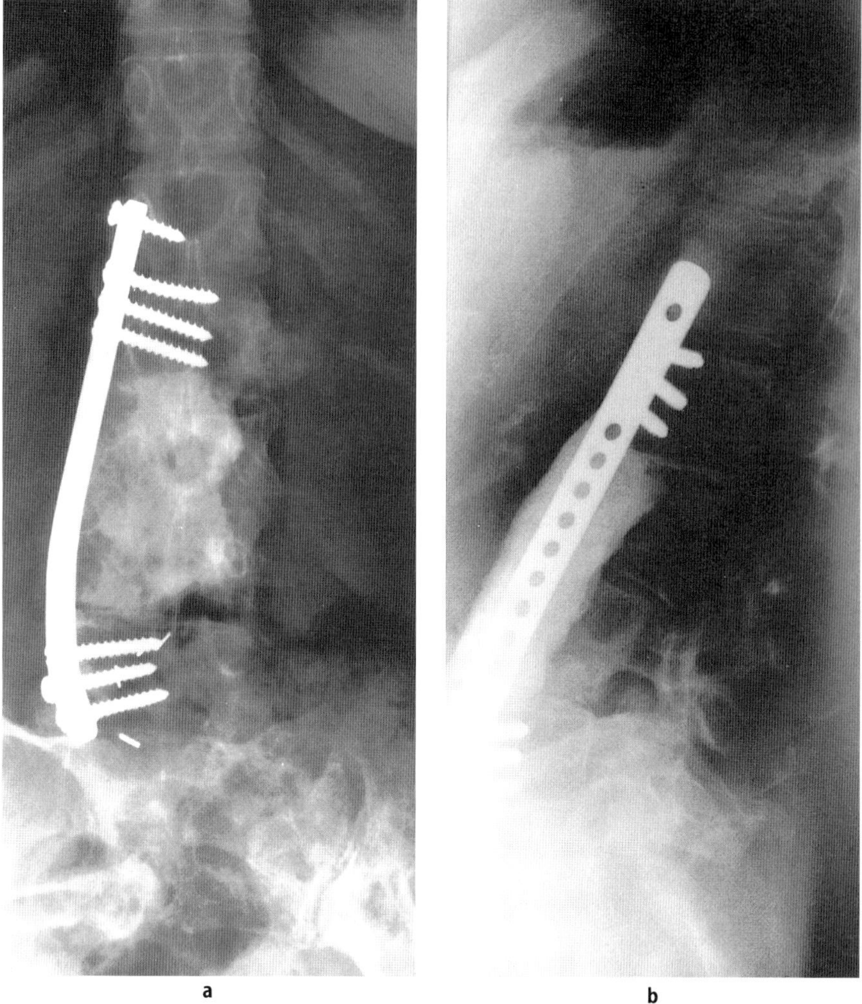

Figure 11.2 L3, L4 vertebral metastases from a breast cancer. Anterior approach with partial excision and stabilisation with cement and plating from L1 to L5. The patient survived for 14 years after the operative procedure

plates with two or three screws in the vertebral body adjacent to the corporectomy, and posteriorly, two screwed pedicular plates for each of the posterior pillars, usually supported on the vertebrae adjacent to the excision (Fig. 11.5). In general, a semi-rigid brace is necessary for 4–6 months.

11.3 Results

Before the advent of vertebral stabilization, only decompressive laminectomy was practised for vertebral metastases, with results no better than those of radiotherapy (Young et al, 1980). Results have improved considerably with the new

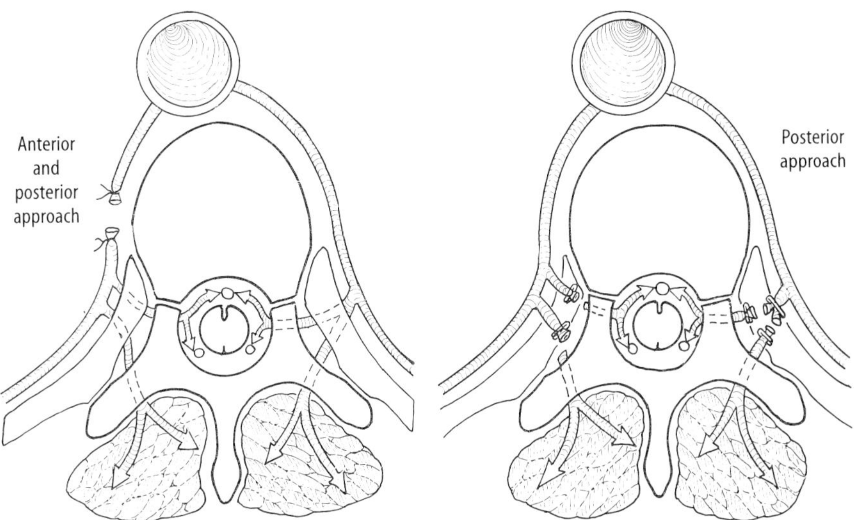

Figure 11.3 Total vertebrectomy using a double anterior and posterior approach (left) and a posterior approach (right). Note the difference in the radiculo-medullary vessels

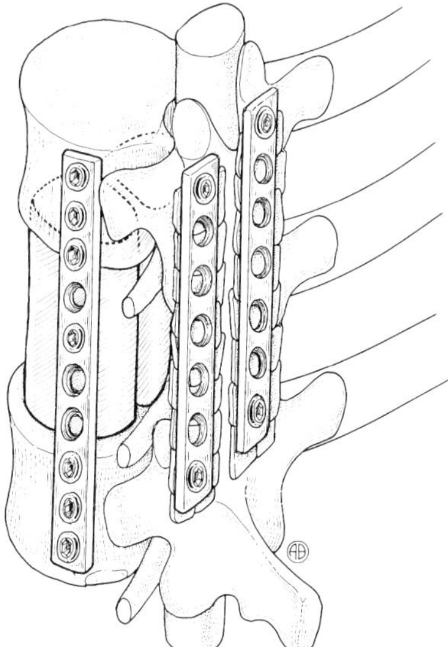

Figure 11.4 Total vertebrectomy with reconstruction of the three pillars using autogenous graft, fibula for the anterior pillar and iliac crest for the two posterior pillars fixed with three plates

anterior or posterior decompression series, combined with stabilization. Siegal (1985) found that 22% of 78 patients could not walk before the operation, while 69% could walk after the operation, an improvement of 54%. The median survival of these patients, after corporectomy, was more than 16 months. Posterior decompression was less effective than anterior decompression.

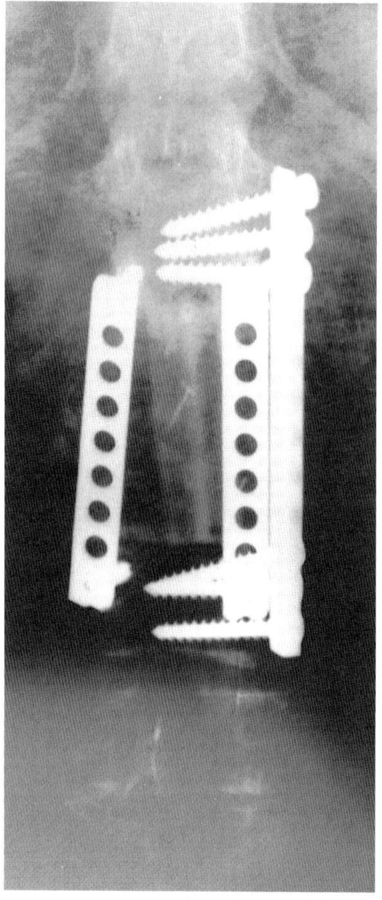

a

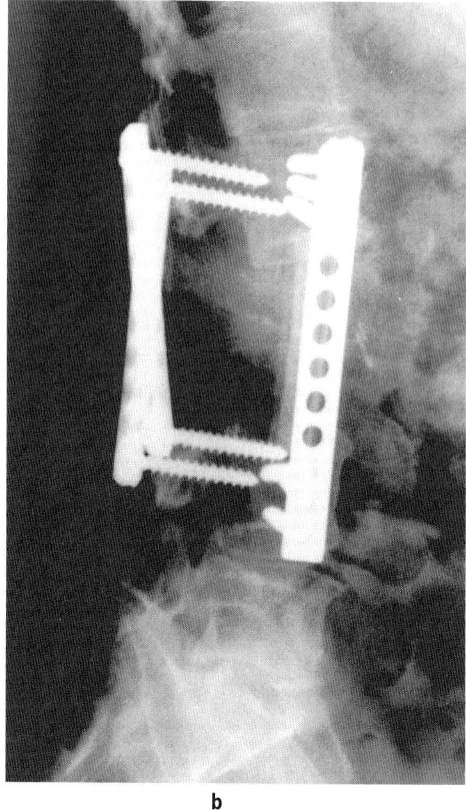

b

Figure 11.5 Total vertebrectomy for L3 metastatic breast cancer. Double approach decompression and stabilisation were performed separately. Two fibular strut grafts were fixed with a plate screwed to the vertebral bodies to reconstruct the anterior pillar and iliac crest graft, with two plates screwed to L2 and L4 pedicles to reconstruct the posterior pillars. The patient regained normal activities and died 34 months later

The results of Nazarian et al (1966) summarise the current state of surgery for vertebral metastases.

11.3.1 The series

A multicentre French study investigated 721 patients who had undergone operations for vertebral metastases. Patients from our department were included in this series. The primitive cancer was breast in 30.4% of cases, unknown in 16%, lung in 13.2%, kidney in 11.7%, prostate in 6.9%, gastrointestinal in 6.7%, thyroid in 5%, uterine in 1.9% and various in 8.3%. The tumour site was isolated to one vertebra in 41.1% and was multivertebral in 33.6% of cases. The tumour was unifocal in 74.7%. Epidural invasion was present in 76.8% of cases. Seventy-three per cent of subjects presented neurological dysfunction, 12% of whom had serious impairment; 55.1% presented no deficit; 11.5% had a sphincter and urinary deficit. Analysis of the results using the Karnofski index showed that 20% of patients were totally autonomous, 46% had limited autonomy and 34% were totally dependent. Only 36.8% of patients had only one vertebral metastasis; 75.2% of patients had no gastrointestinal metastasis.

Preoperative embolisation has been practised in only 15.5% of the patients; 95% of the patients had undergone a limited operation and 5% an extended operation (total vertebrectomy). Among the patients who had a limited operation, 63, 25 and 7% underwent a posterior, anterior and double approach respectively. Blood loss was less than 1 litre, ranged from 1 to 2 litres and was more than 2 litres in 50.3, 35.5 and 13.8% of patients respectively; 62.1% of patients carried a postoperative external support; 42% of patients underwent adjuvant treatment before the operation and 80.7% had postoperative adjuvant treatment.

11.3.2 Global Results

Of patients with preoperative back pain, 19% took only minor pain killers and 91% took major analgesics. At 6 months postoperatively, 81% took minor pain killers, while 19% continued to take major analgesics. Before the operation, 49% of patients took minor pain killers for radiculalgia and 51% took major analgesics. Six months after the operation, 93% took only minor pain killers and 7% major analgesics for radiculalgia. According to the Karnofsky index for physical activity, preoperatively 33% had very reduced activity, 47% had average activity and 20% almost normal activity. At 6 months postoperatively, 12% still had very reduced activity, 38% had average activity and 50% had almost normal activity. Physical performance is therefore improved several months after the operation.

From the neurological point of view, preoperatively 19% of patients were graded Franckel A or B (severe paralysis), 26% C or D and 53% E (normal function). At 6 months postoperatively, 4% were graded A or B, 16% C or D and 80% E. There was therefore a considerable improvement in normal function. The global median survival time was 11 months (11 months postoperatively, 50% of patients were still alive). The median disease-free survival (time after the operation when 50% of the population had no pathological event linked to the cancer) was 7 months in this series. Intraoperative complications included five deaths and postoperatively 6.8% sepsis, 3.9% scar opening, 3% neurological aggravation, 2.6% loosening of the osteosynthesis, 1.6% emboli and 11% local relapses.

11.3.3 Selective Results

The results of limited surgery were not significantly different between the anterior and posterior approaches. Thirty-five of the 721 patients had total vertebrectomy, almost all performed in our department, with particularly good results. At 6 months, 92% of patients were free from back pain and 96% had no more radiculalgia. Seventy per cent have resumed normal activity. From the neurological point of view, of one patient graded Franckel B and three patients graded Franckel C preoperatively, only one patient was graded Franckel C after 6 months, the others having regained almost normal function. The global median survival was 30 months compared with 11 months for limited operations and the median disease-free survival was 20 months compared with 7 months for limited procedures.

11.4 Conclusion

Vertebral stabilization and adjuvant treatment have allowed considerable therapeutic progress over recent decades. The best results are obtained when operations are performed before the patient becomes malnourished and before multiple metastatic sites develop. From the surgical point of view, extended excision as total vertebrectomy gives better results than limited surgery.

References

Batson OV (1940) Function of vertebral veins and their role in spread of metastases. Ann Surg 112:138–149.

Brihaye J, Ectors P, Lemort M et al (1988) The management of spinal epidural metastases. Adv Tech Stand Neurosurg 16:121.

Deramond H, Debussche C, Pruvo JP et al (1990) La vertébroplastie. Feuillets de Radiologie 30:262–268.

De Wald RL, Bridwell KH, Prodromas C et al (1985) Reconstructive spinal surgery as palliation of metastatic malignancies of the spine. Spine 10(1):21–26.

Louis R (1983) Surgery of the spine. Surgical anatomy and operative approaches. Springer-Verlag, Berlin.

Nazarian S et al (1997) Symposium: place de la chirurgie dans le traitement des métastases du rachis. SOFCOT 1996. Rev Chir Orthop 83(suppl III):109–174.

Roy-Camille R, Saillant G, Lapresle P et al (1985) Surgical treatment of spinal metastases by stabilization using plates screwed into the vertebral pedicles. Rev Chir Orthop 71(7):483.

Siegal T (1985) Surgical decompression of anterior and posterior malignant epidural tumours compressing the spinal cord: a prospective study. Neurosurgery 17(3):424.

Tokuhashi Y, Matsuzaki H, Toriyama S et al (1990) Scoring system for the preoperative evaluation of metastatic spine tumour prognosis. Spine 15:1110–1113.

Wong DA, Fornasier VL, McNab I (1990) Spinal metastases: the obvious, the occult and the impostors. Spine 15:1–4.

Young RF, Post EM, King GA (1980) Treatment of spinal epidural metastases. Randomized prospective comparison of laminectomy and radiotherapy. J Neurosurg 53(6):741.

Further Reading

Asdourian PL (1991) Metastatic disease of the spine In: Bridwell KH, De Wald RL (eds) Textbook of spinal surgery. JB Lippincott, Philadelphia.

Clark CR, Keggi KJ, Panjabi M (1984) Methylmethacrylate stabilization of the cervical spine. J Bone Joint Surg 66A(1):40.

Crock HV, Yoshizawa H, Kame SK (1973) Observation on the veinous drainage of the human vertebral body. J Bone Joint Surg 54:528–533.

Findlay G (1987) The role of vertebral body collapse in the management of malignant spinal cord compression. J Neurol Neurosurg Psychiatr 50:151–154.

Galasko CSB (1976) Relations of bone distribution in skeletal mestastases to osteoclast activation and prostaglandins. Nature 263:508–510.

Harrington KD (1981) The use of methylmethacrylate for vertebral-body replacement and anterior stabilization of pathological fracture-dislocations of the spine due to metastatic malignant disease. J Bone Joint Surg 63A(1):36–46.

Harrington KD (1984) Anterior cord decompression and spinal stabilization for patients with metastatic lesions of the spine. J Neurosurg 61(1):107.

Kostuik JP (1983) Anterior spinal cord decompression for lesions of the thoracic and lumbar spine techniques, new methods of internal fixation results. Spine 8(5):512.

Onimus M, Laurain JM (1991) Histoire naturelle des métastases vertébrales. Deuxièmes Journées d'Orthopédie de l'Hôpital Saint-Jacques, 7 et 8 mai, Besanc[,]on.

White WA, Patterson RH Jr, Bergland RM (1971) Role of surgery in the treatment of spinal cord compression by metastatic neoplasm. Cancer 27(3):558.

12 Treatment of Secondary Spinal Tumours

C.S.B. Galasko and J.B. Spilsbury

12.1 Introduction

The diagnosis and treatment of spinal metastatic tumours is an increasing part of an orthopaedic spinal surgeon's role, as the life expectancy of patients with treatable malignancy increases.

The spine is the most common site of skeletal metastasis; 60% of all skeletal lesions and 36% of all vertebral lesions are asymptomatic and discovered incidentally. Symptomatic spinal column involvement occurs in approximately 18,000 patients per year in the USA and 9000 in Britain. According to Brihaye et al (1988), 15% of tumours metastasising to the spine were from the lung, 16.5% from the breast, 6.5% from the kidney, 9.2% from the thyroid, gastrointestinal tract 4.6%, miscellaneous 10.8%, and unknown 5%. Seventy per cent of metastasis in the spine occurred in the thoracic and thoracolumbar region, 21% in the lumbosacral region, and 8% in the cervical and cervicothoracic region.

Traditionally, metastatic tumours involving the spine have been treated palliatively with increasing opiate-based analgesics, etc. Over the past two decades, however, there has been a growing interest in the surgical management of these patients, with an aim of stabilisation of the spine and decompression of the spinal cord where appropriate in order to increase the patient's quality of life, and reduce their analgesic requirements. The basis of oncologic spinal surgery is, in the vast majority of cases, still palliative treatment, as even total resection of a metastatic lesion will not affect outcome, which is usually determined by other secondaries. The aim of surgery in all cases is to increase the patient's mobility, reduce their pain and preserve bladder and bowel function, thus overall increasing their quality of life.

The biomechanics of the normal spine have been well described. Studies performed by Harms demonstrated approximately 80% of the forces through the spinal column are transmitted through the anterior column, i.e. through the disc and vertebral bodies (Lowery and Harms, 1997). Secondary deposits are more common in the vertebral body as opposed to the posterior elements, and this predisposes to kyphotic collapse, as the metastatic tissue is structurally less able to transmit these forces than normal cancellous bone.

12.2 Consideration of the Primary Tumour

Before making a treatment plan, it is important that the histopathological diagnosis is made. This requires biopsy. Biopsy can be performed either transpedicularly, or with a suitable needle percutaneously under computed tomography-guided control. It is important wherever possible to make a tissue diagnosis before planning treatment, as prognosis depends on the primary tumour.

12.2.1 Breast

The primary tumour most commonly treated by spinal surgeons originates from the breast. At post-mortem, approximately 85% of patients with breast cancer had skeletal metastasis. The spine is involved in between 19 and 70% of patients. A solitary bone metastasis is the initial sign of recurrent disease in 21% of patients and 52% of solitary metastases are within the spine. Between 2 and 12.5% of patients with spinal metastasis develop neurological deterioration. The prognosis for breast cancer is improving with more aggressive chemotherapy. With a more proactive approach to metastatic breast carcinoma, younger patients are now being referred for treatment.

12.2.2 Prostate

Prostate cancer is found in post-mortem specimens, in between 24 and 46% of men over the age of 50 years. Prostate cancer commonly metastasises to bone, and commonly occurs in the thoracic spine. Most prostate cancer can be treated hormonally; the prognosis for life expectancy when cord compression occurs is better than for most other tumours. Like multiple myeloma, life expectancy can be measured in years, if the tumour can be controlled by pharmacological means.

12.2.3 Myeloma

Myeloma is one of the commonest tumours involving the spine in men. The prognosis for myeloma is good as far as life expectancy is concerned, as myeloma can often be satisfactorily treated with chemotherapy and radiotherapy. For this reason, tumours involving compression of the cord should be treated aggressively, with early surgery. Bone grafting is important, as the patient will often survive long enough for implant failure to occur unless an adequate fusion is achieved.

12.2.4 Other Primary Tumours

Primary tumours from the lung usually require only palliative treatment as life expectancy is often no more than a few months. There are occasional exceptions to this and guidance from an oncologist and histopathologist is required before a treatment plan is made. Renal cell carcinoma is a specific problem, as these tumours are often very vascular. If it is not recognised before surgery that a renal cell tumour is present, the patient may exsanguinate during the surgical procedure. Before definitive surgery, embolisation of the tumour significantly reduces the vascularity and therefore is indicated in all renal cell tumours.

12.2.5 Bone Graft

When spinal instrumentation is undertaken, bone grafting is essential in patients with a "normal" life expectancy. This is because spinal implants fatigue when under continuous load and all implants will eventually fail, unless an adequate fusion takes place. However in oncology patients, achievement of fusion is not essential, as life expectancy is short, often being less than a year. In cases where life expectancy is limited, bone graft is not necessary. In this case our preferred method is to pack the cage with cement. This increases the strength of the cage to compressive forces and acts as a space filler. Where survival is thought to be longer than a year, we attempt anterior fusion. In this case, the harvesting of autologous bone graft is contraindicated. This is for two reasons:

- The pelvis may be a site of metastasis or micrometastasis. To insert this into the cage would be inappropriate
- Posterior iliac crest bone graft may be a source of constant pain postoperatively, which is best avoided if possible.

Allograft or bone substitute is packed in and around the cage to enhance fusion.

12.2.6 Patient Selection

Not all patients are suitable for anterior surgery, because of the widespread nature of their metastasis, the poor prognosis of their primary tumour, or the poor medical fitness of the patient for major surgery. All patients require full staging before surgery. Our own protocol includes magnetic resonance imaging of the whole spine (to rule out other spinal lesions), bone scan, ultrasound of abdomen, chest radiograph and full hematological work-up. Tokuhashi et al (1994) has made an attempt at a scoring system in order to guide as to whether palliative stabilisation or more radical palliative resection should be undertaken. The Tokuhashi score attempts to segregate those who would benefit from anterior surgery and those who would benefit from posterior stabilisation alone. It is a useful tool but has not been fully validated and is only a guide to selection. The Karnofski score is a functional score, which can be used to assess changes in outcome following major surgery for spinal metastasis.

12.3 Surgery

12.3.1 Indications for Surgery

There are two prime indications for surgery in patients with metastatic cancer: spinal instability and compression of the spinal cord or cauda equina.

12.3.1.1 Spinal Instability

Back pain is a frequent symptom of disseminated cancer and in 10% of patients with spinal metastasis is due to spinal instability (Galasko and Sylvester, 1978). There are two causes for spinal instability in metastatic cancer: bone destruction due to the tumour and iatrogenic. The latter occurs following a posterior decompression for a cord/cauda equina compression without simultaneous stabilisation. Spinal instability can cause excruciating pain that is mechanical in nature. In its severe form the patient is comfortable only when lying absolutely still and any movement, including log rolling by two or three trained nurses, may be associated with agonising pain. The patient may be unable to sit, stand or walk because of the pain, even with the use of a spinal orthosis. Plain radiographs show destruction of bone with vertebral collapse of a greater or lesser degree. It is unusual for a discrete fracture to be seen but, nevertheless, spinal instability should be considered the equivalent of a pathological fracture in a long bone, because the pain is due to the instability and not the metastasis. Radiotherapy, chemotherapy or endocrine therapy, even if successful in controlling the tumour, will not alleviate the pain. Like pathological fractures of the long bones, stabilisation is required for pain relief.

The spine can be stabilised by either a posterior or anterior approach (Bridwell et al, 1988; Cybulski, 1989; De Wald et al, 1985; Fidler, 1987, 1994; Flatley et al, 1984; Galasko, 1991; Harrington, 1981; Hertlein et al, 1992; Hosono et al, 1995).

12.3.1.2 Compression of the Spinal Cord or Cauda Equina

Schaberg and Gainor (1985) reported that cord compression occurred in 20% of patients with vertebral metastases. Constans et al (1983) thought it likely that 5–10% of patients with spinal metastasis developed symptomatic neurological manifestations of their metastases. Compression of the spinal cord or cauda equina may occur in association with spinal instability (where the treatment of choice is spinal stabilisation, decompression and postoperative radiotherapy) or in isolation. In the latter circumstance, the choice of treatment depends on the duration, severity and rapidity of onset of the symptoms. Pain is almost invariable and persisting and increasing back pain may herald spinal cord compression. The pain is frequently localised to the site of the disease and is probably caused by stimulation of pain receptors in the longitudinal ligaments, dura or periosteum as the tumour expands. Radicular pain is less common. Nevertheless, by the time treatment is started, up to 50% of patients will no longer be able to walk and 10–30% will be paraplegic (Galasko, 1986; Fidler, 1987).

Other symptoms include weakness, disturbance of gait, paraesthesia, urinary hesitancy or precipitance and constipation or spurious diarrhoea. The sequence of events is often pain, motor dysfunction, paraesthesia and sensory loss. The results depend heavily on the neurological status of the patient at the time of starting treatment and it is important, therefore, to make the diagnosis urgently. Surgery is indicated in patients with: recent onset of symptoms, particularly a developing paraplegia or urinary retention of less than 24 hours' duration; a block shown on the preoperative magnetic resonance image, localised to no more than two or three segments; and a life expectancy of least 2–3 months. Once paraplegia has been established for some days, or urinary retention has been present for more than 24–30 hours, surgery is often associated with some return of sensation and/or pain relief, but not with useful recovery of bladder or motor functions.

Occasionally, anterior decompression and stabilisation may be associated with major neurological recovery in patients with longstanding neurological disturbances where the onset of the symptoms has been gradual. In general terms, patients with a gradual onset of neurological disturbances do better than those who have developed paraplegia and urinary retention extremely rapidly. Decompression should never be carried out without simultaneous stabilisation. Laminectomy alone is contraindicated. It leads to increased instability of the spine. Studies that compare laminectomy and radiotherapy with radiotherapy alone are flawed, in that they are comparing a destabilising operation with radiotherapy. Decompression and stabilisation may be either posterior or anterior (see below). Treatment should also be combined with a short course of high-dose steroids to minimise the oedema. Laminectomy without stabilisation will often cause further instability with increasing kyphosis, increasing pain and increased neurological deficit.

O'Donoghue et al (1997) found that in patients with structurally significant bone destruction secondary to metastases from breast cancer, surgery and radiotherapy were associated with a speedier resolution of symptoms, a longer symptom-free survival, a lower incidence of symptom recurrence and a longer survival overall than radiotherapy alone. The symptom-free survival in patients with structurally significant bone destruction of their axial skeleton was 11 weeks in patients treated with radiotherapy alone compared with 39 weeks in patients treated with surgery and radiotherapy ($p<0.5$). The overall survival in these patients was 9.4 months in those treated with radiotherapy alone, compared with 22.3 months in those treated with surgery and radiotherapy ($p<0.05$).

12.3.2 Posterior Stabilisation

Posterior stabilisation has been practised for many years. It is a more straightforward approach surgically, being less invasive to the patient. The approach is well known by most orthopaedic surgeons, instrumentation is relatively straightforward, and postoperative management of such patients requires less monitoring and is less intensive. Posterior stabilisation is usually less of a surgical insult to the patient and therefore such surgery can be performed on less medically fit patients. As has already been discussed, most of the metastatic deposits are anterior, and therefore the posterior structures at the level of pathology are relatively strong, consisting of pedicles and laminae unaffected by the disease process. If stabilisation is combined with a decompressive procedure, these relatively intact structures (spinous processes, interspinous ligaments and laminae) require removal for the indirect decompression to be undertaken. Thus, in a posterior decompression, the spine is destabilised further by sacrificing intact bony elements to decompress indirectly the neural elements.

Posterior decompression alone, without stabilisation, is contraindicated because of the further destabilising effect. If a posterior decompression is felt appropriate, it should **always** be combined with posterior instrumentation in order to restore stability. It is usually possible, when performing a posterior stabilisation, to use pedicle screws, sublaminar hooks, or sublaminar wires. However, implant failure will occur, either by implant breakage or implant pull out, unless either a sound bony fusion occurs, or the patient succumbs to the malignancy. Posterior stabilisation is also mechanically inferior as the deficient anterior column is not reconstructed. Therefore force has to be transferred to the posterior elements. At least two spinal segments must be stabilised on each side of the pathological level, so in total five levels or more require instrumentation when combined with a one-level posterior decompression (Figs 12.1–12.3).

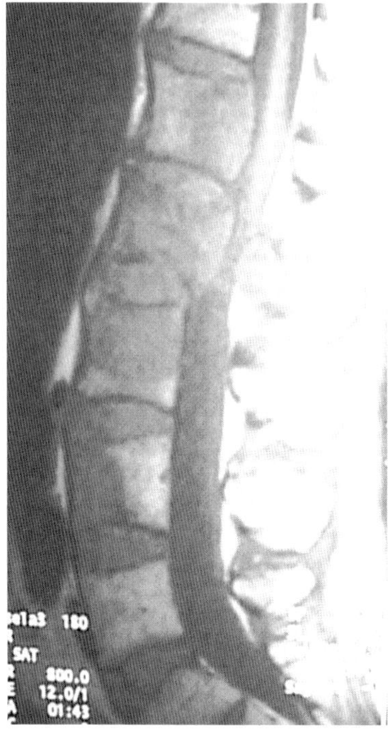

Figure 12.1 Magnetic resonance image of a 71-year-old man with multiple spinal metastases from the prostate. He presented with Grade 3 power in his legs. The scan reveals cord compression at L1 and L2, with metastases in L1, L2, L3 and L4

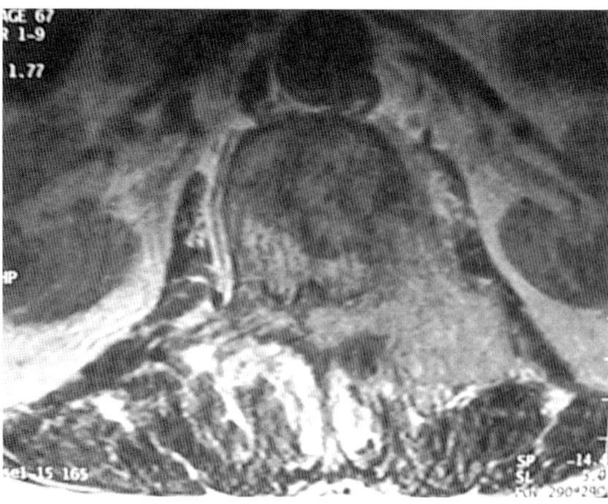

Figure 12.2 Significant posterior compression in the patient shown in Fig. 12.1

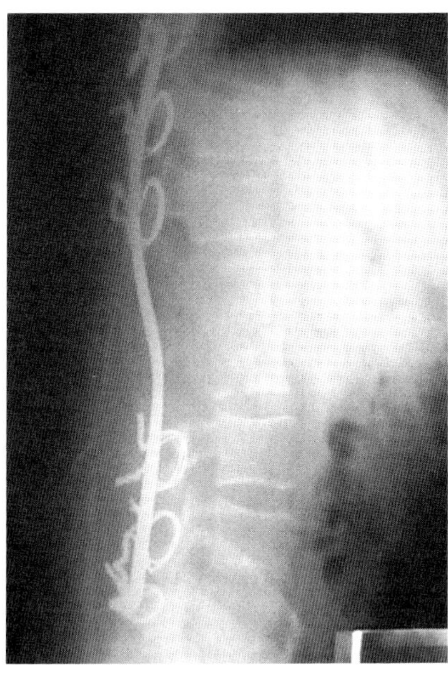

Figure 12.3 Postoperative X-ray following multiple-level stabilisation with L1 and L2 posterior decompression. The patient's neurology significantly improved and his instability pain settled. Adjuvant therapy was necessary

In summary, we believe that posterior surgery has a number of drawbacks when compared with anterior surgery:

- The indirect decompression may be inferior, as the compression is anterior to neural elements
- The decompression performed posteriorly destabilises the spine further, making instrumentation necessary
- A long construct is necessary to achieve stability, but without anterior column reconstruction this is mechanically inferior.

12.3.3 Anterior Decompression and Stabilisation

Anterior decompression and stabilisation (Johnson et al, 1983) has more recently become the approach of choice when treating neurological compression. This is because it allows direct decompression and stabilisation, restoring anterior column function and allowing a better biomechanical reconstruction.

The anterior approach to the spine was first employed by Hodgson et al (1960) and has become known as the Hong Kong technique, for the debridement of tuberculous vertebral osteomyelitis. It has only recently become widely used to decompress tumours because it is a more demanding technique, requiring more intensive monitoring of the patient and more sophisticated anaesthetic techniques.

The thoracic spine can be exposed anteriorly with ease through a right thoracotomy exposing up to T5 to allow vertebrectomy. However, reconstruction anteriorly with screw and rod systems (Kaneda or Ventrafix type device) is not indicated at this level, as this would involve screws into T4, which are contra-indicated because of metalwork close to the great vessels. At this level in the spine, vertebrectomy can be performed, with additional posterior stabilisation with hooks or pedicle screws to secure the cage. The rest of the thoracic spine can easily be approached to allow a full corporectomy and stabilisation using the Kaneda device with bicortical screws to allow secure fixation (Kaneda et al, 1997). The posterior longitudinal ligament is visualised and well decompressed, an appropriate-sized titanium mesh cage can be inserted to restore vertebral height (therefore reducing the kyphosis and allowing restoration of anterior column support) and compression of adjacent vertebral bodies with the Kaneda device concludes the reconstruction.

Anterior stabilisation requires normal bone-quality cephalad and caudad to the level of vertebrectomy, in order to obtain secure fixation. Multiple level vertebral metastases (even when they do not cause compression) interfere with secure fixation, and are therefore a relative contraindication to anterior vertebrectomy. Severe osteoporosis is also a relative contraindication, as construction failure (by cage sinkage or screw pull out) can occur. Surgery in the lumbar region can be performed with relative ease using a left retroperitoneal approach. An L4 vertebrectomy is surgically more demanding, and often requires posterior stabilisation with pedicle screws, as it is difficult to instrument L5 because of the proximity of the great vessels. An L5 vertebrectomy also has unique problems. It is usually not possible to insert an anterior screw into S1, and therefore posterior stabilisation is necessary. If an L5 vertebrectomy is to be performed, this may perhaps be easiest through a transperitoneal approach, though a retroperitoneal approach is also possible (Figs 12.4–12.6).

More recently, endoscopically assisted decompression has been undertaken (McLain, 1998). McLain's conclusion was that endoscopic-assisted decompression

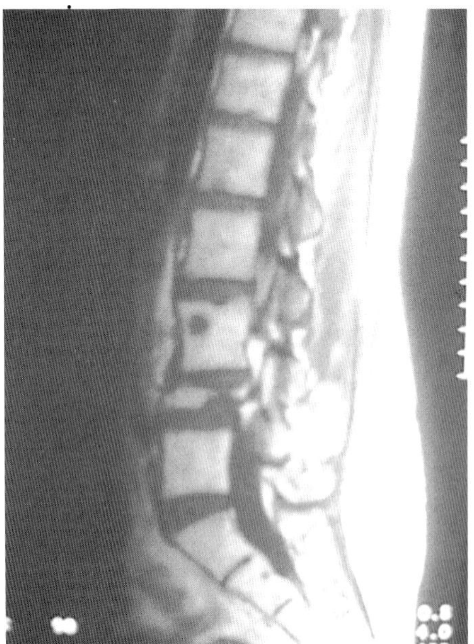

Figure 12.4 Magnetic resonance image of a 38-year-old woman with cancer of the breast and collapse of L4 and tumour in L3

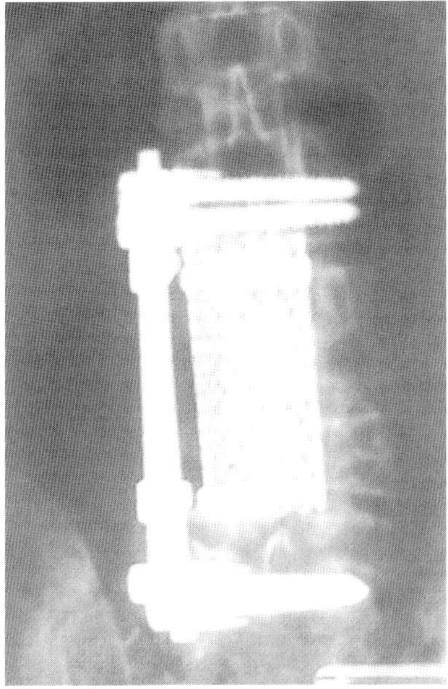

Figure 12.5 Postoperative X-ray of the woman shown in Fig. 12.4

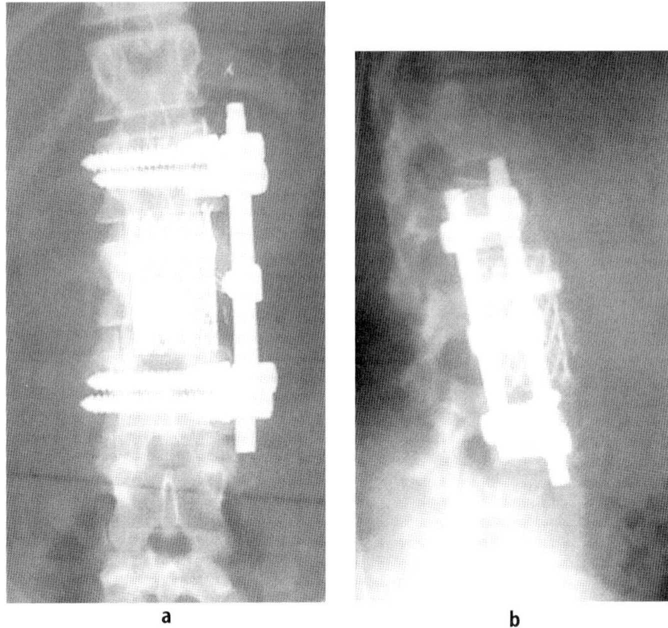

Figure 12.6 X-rays 6 months following L2 vertebrectomy for breast metastasis

can reduce morbidity, and may aid surgery, improving the surgeon's vision, providing light and magnification as well as a more direct view. We have no personal experience of thoracoscopic vertebrectomy.

12.3.4 Combined Anterior and Posterior Surgery

Occasionally, paraplegia, or impending paraplegia, is caused by circumferential tumour. In this case, anterior and posterior stabilisation will give the best palliative approach, allowing debulking of tumour from both anterior and posterior approaches, with rigid stabilisation. It is our own preference, wherever possible, to perform anterior decompression and stabilisation alone. However, where there is significant posterior tumour that requires decompression, and/or osteoporosis, which would increase the risk of anterior construct failure, anterior decompression is supplemented by posterior stabilisation (Figs 12.7 and 12.8).

12.3.5 Results of our own Series

We now have 23 patients (eight males and 15 females, age range 37–85 years) who are over a year post anterior vertebrectomy, Moss cage and Kaneda device. Their mean age at surgery was 55 years 8 months. The most common primary tumour in women was breast (eight) and in men myeloma (four). Karnofski scores ranged from 57% preoperatively (range 30–80%) to 85% postoperatively (range 70–90%). This calculates to a change in Karnofski score of 27%, which equates to most patients becoming independent, whereas previously they were dependent for most activities of daily living. No patients deteriorated neurologically, 62% started at Franckel E, where they remained, 30% improved from Franckel D to Franckel E and one patient improved from Franckel C to Franckel E. There was a marked decrease in the consumption of opiates and analgesics after the operation (V. Lykomitros, J. Spilsbury, R. Ross, J. Williamson, submitted for publication).

In an earlier study (Galasko et al 2000), we reported on 80 patients with spinal instability who had been treated by a variety of methods of stabilisation. Five patients were treated by anterior stabilisation, five by combined anterior and posterior stabilisation and 70 by posterior stabilisation alone, using a variety of types of instrumentation. Eighty-nine per cent of patients obtained complete relief of pain and 5% partial relief of pain. Thirty-four of the 80 patients had clinical evidence of compression of their spinal cord or cauda equina, usually weakness of the lower limbs severe enough to affect walking or standing and sometimes associated with loss of bladder function. These patients were treated by decompression at the time of stabilisation. Of the 34 patients, 23 (68%) obtained major recovery of neurological function sufficient to allow them to walk without orthoses and to restore bladder function where it had been compromised. In two patients, cord compression recurred 10 and 14 months, respectively, after decompression. Onimus et al (1996) has reported similar results.

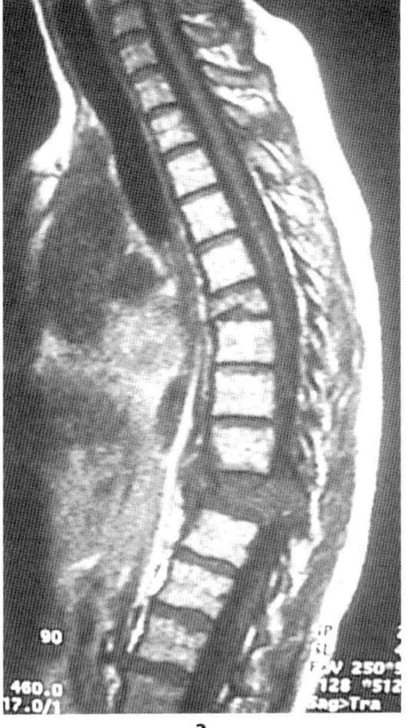

a

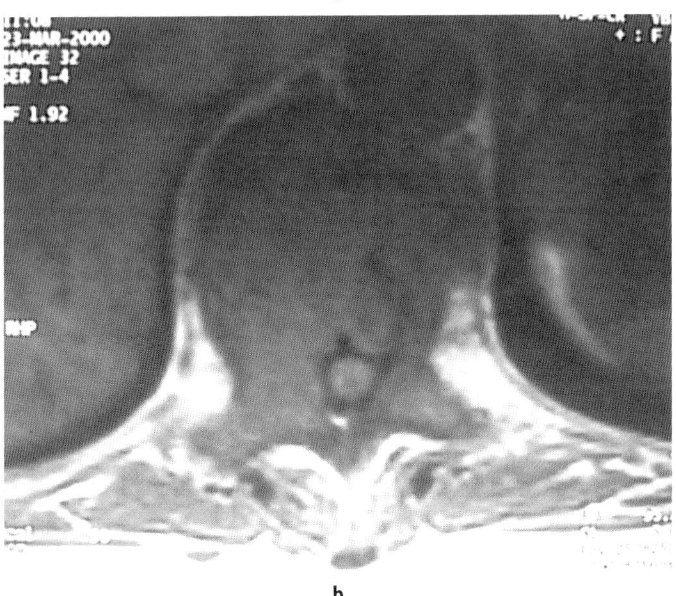

b

Figure 12.7 Magnetic resonance image of a 53-year-old woman with T10 circumferential cord compression, presenting with right-sided thoracic radicular pain and instability. Primary tumour breast. Note collapse of T6 from metastasis treated 2 years earlier with radiotherapy

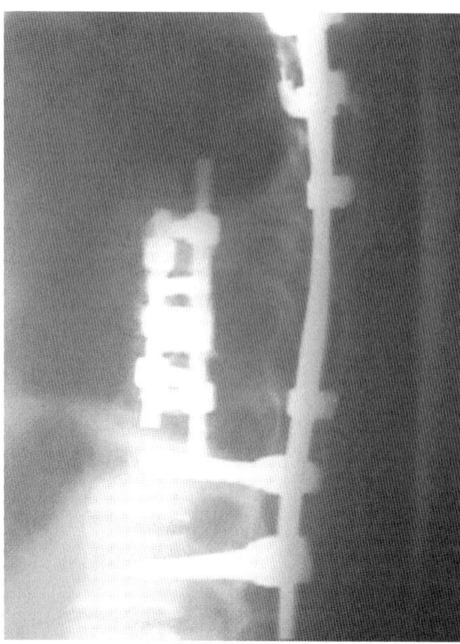

Figure 12.8 Postoperative X-ray showing front and back T10 vertebrectomy, Kaneda device and Moss cage plus sequential posterior Isola construct, with eight hooks proximally and four pedicle screws distally, with posterior decompression of the tumour at T10 and T11

12.4 Vertebroplasty

Vertebroplasty is a further way of stabilising a spine in a minimally invasive way (Cotten et al, 1996; Cunin et al, 2000; Einhorn, 2000). It involves the percutaneous injection of bone cement into lytic lesions in the vertebral body in order to provide support and prevent collapse of the vertebral body. Basically, it takes advantage of interventional radiological techniques. It has been used in the treatment of osteolytic lesions, including myeloma and spinal metastases (Weill et al, 1996). Despite the number of articles published on this procedure, few have clearly defined the outcome measures and virtually none have provided a long-term follow-up, in terms of the clinical indications, expected complications and inherent risks. What happens with time?

12.5 Conclusion

Treatment of metastatic spinal disease is a complex process. It involves a team of oncologists and radiotherapists, histopathologists, skilled anesthetists, radiologists, spinal surgeons and dedicated nursing staff. Treatment often involves palliative decompression and stabilisation, followed by further oncological treatment with chemotherapy and radiotherapy. For long-term survival, control of the tumour is essential. Advances in implant design and surgical techniques have allowed a more aggressive approach to these tumours, with rewarding results. However, patient selection is still difficult and requires a team approach.

References

Bridwell KH, Jenny AB, Saul T et al (1988) Posterior segmental spinal instrumentation (PSSI) with posterolateral decompression and debulking for metastatic thoracic and lumbar spine disease: limitations of the technique. Spine 13:1383–1394.
Brihaye J, Ectors P, Lemort M et al (1988) The management of spinal epidural metastases. Adv Tech Stand Neurosurg 16:121.
Constans JP, de Divitiis E, Donzelli R et al (1983) Spinal metastases with neurological manifestations. Review of 600 cases. J Neurosurg 59:111–118.
Cotten A, Dewatre F, Cortet B et al (1996) Percutaneous vertebroplasty for osteolytic metastases and myeloma: effects of the percentage of lesion filling and the leakage of methyl methacrylate at clinical follow-up. Radiology 200:525–530.
Cunin G, Boissonnett H, Petite H et al (2000) Experimental vertebroplasty using osteoconductive granular material. Spine 25:1070–1076.
Cybulski GR (1989) Methods of surgical stabilisation of metastatic disease of the spine. Neurosurgery 25:240–252.
De Wald RL, Bridwell KH, Prodromas C et al (1985) Reconstructive spinal surgery as palliation of metastatic malignancies of the spine. Spine 10(1):21–26.
Einhorn TA (2000) Vertebroplasty: an opportunity to do something really good for patients. Spine 25:1051–1052.
Fidler MW (1987) Pathological fractures of the spine including those causing anterior spinal cord compression: surgical management. In: Galasko CSB, Noble J (eds) Recent developments in orthopaedic surgery; Festschrift to Sir Harry Platt. Manchester University Press, Manchester, pp 94–103.
Fidler MW (1994) Radical resection of vertebral body tumours: a surgical technique used in ten cases. J Bone Joint Surg Br 76:765–772.
Flatley TJ, Anderson MH, Anast GY (1984) Spinal instability due to malignant disease: treatment by segmental spinal stabilisation. J Bone Joint Surg Am 66:47–52.
Galasko CSB (1986) Skeletal metastases. Butterworth, London.
Galasko CSB (1991) Spinal instability secondary to metastatic cancer. J Bone Joint Surg Br 73:104–108.
Galasko CSB, Norris HE, Crank S (2000) Spinal instability secondary to metastatic cancer. J Bone Joint Surg 82A:570–576.
Galasko CSB, Sylvester BS (1978) Back pain in patients treated for malignant tumours. Clin Oncol 4:273–283.
Harrington KD (1981) The use of methylmethacrylate for vertebral-body replacement and anterior stabilization of pathological fracture-dislocations of the spine due to metastatic malignant disease. J Bone Joint Surg 63A(1):36–46.
Hertlein H, Mittlmeier T, Piltz S et al (1992) Spinal stabilisation for patients with metastatic lesions of the spine using a titanium spacer. Eur Spine J 1:131–136.
Hodgson AR, Stock FF, Yang HS et al (1960) Anterior spinal fusion. The operative approach and pathological findings in 412 patients with Potts disease of the spine. Br J Surg 48:172.
Hosono N, Yonenobu K, Fuji T et al (1995) Orthopaedic management of spinal metastases. Clin Orthop 312:148–159.
Johnson JR, Leatherman KD, Holt RT (1983) Anterior decompression of the spinal cord for neurological deficit. Spine 8:396–405.
Kaneda K, Taneichi H, Abumi K et al (1997) Anterior decompression and stabilisation with the Kaneda device for thoraco-lumbar burst fractures associated with neurological deficits. J Bone Joint Surg Am 79A:69–83.
Lowery GL, Harms J (1997) Principles of load sharing. In: Bridwell KH, De Wald RL (eds) Textbook of spinal surgery, 2nd edn, ch 13. Lippincott-Raven, Philadelphia.
McLain RF (1998) Endoscopically assisted compression of metastatic thoracic neoplasms. Spine 23:113–235.
O'Donoghue DS, Howell A, Walls J (1997) Orthopaedic management of structurally significant bone destruction in breast cancer bone metastasis. In the Proceedings of the British Orthopaedic Association. J Bone Joint Surg 79B(suppl 1):98.
Onimus M, Pappin P, Ganlough F (1996) Results of surgical treatment of spinal thoracic and lumbar metastasis. Eur Spine J 5:407–411.
Schaberg J, Gainor BJ (1985) A profile of metastatic carcinoma of the spine. Spine 10:19–20.

Tokuhashi Y, Matzaki H, Kawano H et al (1994) The indication of operative procedure for a metastatic spine tumor: a scoring system for the pre-operative evaluation of the prognosis. J Japan Orthopaed Assoc 68:379–389.

Weill A, Chiras J, Simon JM et al (1996) Spinal metastases: indications for and results of percutaneous injection of acrylic surgical cement. Radiol 199:241–247.

Further Reading

Belkoff SM, Mathis JM, Erbe EM et al (2000) Biomechanical evaluation of a new bone cement for use in vertebroplasty. Spine 25:1061–1064.

Boxer BI, Todd CE, Coleman R et al (1989) Bone secondaries in breast cancer: the solitary metastasis. J Nucl Med 30:1318.

Findley GF (1984) Adverse effects of the management of spinal cord compression. J Neurol Neurosurg Psychiat 47:761–768.

Galasko CSB (1996) Mechanisms of bone destruction in the development of skeletal metastasis. Nature 263(5577):507.

Gurr KE, McAffee PC, Shih CM (1988) Biomechanical analysis of anterior and posterior instrumentation systems after corpectomy. J Bone Joint Surg 70A:1182.

Kanayama M, Ng JT, Cunningham BW et al (1999) Biomechanical analysis of anterior versus circumferential spinal reconstruction for various anatomic stages of tumor lesions. Spine 24(5):445–450.

McLain RF, Sparling E, Benson DR (1993) Early failure of short segment pedicle instrumentation for thoraco lumbar fractures. J Bone Joint Surg 75:162.

Part 6

Medico-social Aspects

13 Caring for Cancer Patients

D. Chevassut

13.1 Introduction

For several years, I have been teaching caregivers how to meet the needs of patients suffering from cancer or from other severe pathology, within the Public Assistance of Marseille.

Three main themes have appeared in classifying the expectations and motivations of the health professionals who have participated in this training. In order of frequency, they are as follows:

- How to find an adequate attitude (knowing what to say, knowing what to do) when facing suffering and death of others
- How to help others efficiently without destroying oneself
- How to accept the reality of suffering and death and become less scared of them.

After several years and many progressive evaluations, we became acutely aware of the necessity to emphasise obvious, often painful and usually forgotten realities that are indispensable for the "right" caring of suffering people. Reminding caregivers of these fundamental notions seems to have helped many to improve the quality of their relationship with the suffering patient, the latter obtaining a secondary non-neglectful benefit from it. These simple realities are concerned, on one hand, with general reflection on life, birth and death; on the other hand, with a more global approach of what is usually called a "human being".

It is surprising to see how an atmosphere of confusion and forgetting these profound truths might result in an additional source of suffering, indeed tragedies.

13.2 Life, Birth and Death

The word "life" has several meanings. Life has many aspects, but three points are essential when discussing human suffering and death. Reflection on and awareness of these points lead to a more profound, relaxed and serene vision of the problem:

- Life as existence
- Life as inner unity and idea that provides a direction
- Life as a dynamic force, energy, or vitality and creative principle.

13.2.1 Life as Existence

Life as existence is limited in time and space. It is the human existence with all that is implied in happiness and suffering. It is life as duration and quality. It is the apparent part of life.

13.2.2 Life as Inner Unity and Idea that Provides a Direction

This manifests itself and is expressed according to a coherent organisation; it is life as a principle of information or organisation power.

Imagine a centre and a periphery: the periphery is precisely organised and structured in relation to the centre. The nature and quality of the centre influence and give form to a manifested environment. This law of life is expressed in many fields, whether it is in the organisation of nature or society. In a hospital unit, for example, the head of the unit, who is the central pillar of the medical team, often creates dynamics and habits that are his or her own. The unit is entirely organised around the dynamics created by the centre. This also relates to the environment that surrounds the patient.

However, life also structures and organises, alternating in a constructive or destructive manner. It is easy to conceive the constructive aspect of life, but harder to conceive its destructive aspect. For example, theories on ageing suggest a kind of genetic programming of the cells. At the time of fertilisation, the egg and cells that stem from it are already programmed to age and die. We can say that the acceptance of death by the cell allows the evolution of the total structure. A cancerous cell that proliferates in an anarchical way and that does not want to die, endangers the entire system to which it belongs.

In reality, all things in the formation of nature also apply to human beings as one of the components of nature.

Life is made up of cycles of births and deaths, and of an alternation of births and deaths. Birth and death are an integral part of life and their alternation maintains, in some ways, the process of life. We can even formulate the following equation: Life = Birth × Death.

Presentation of this equation, although imperfect, is interesting, because it shows that a human being who denies the reality of death in day-to-day life has many difficulties living. Seen in a certain perspective, the fear of dying is as revealing as the fear of living. It is the "sacrifice" of the cell that permits life to flow totally without impediment. This is also the profound and sacred meaning of death. Similarly, a society that denies death will lose the meaning of sacred and simply the meaning of life. Sacred therefore implies the respect of birth and death, of the structuring and destructuring. From this perspective, we obtain an insight into some types of risky or suicidal behaviour observed nowadays, such as extreme sports and drug addiction. Flirting with death is fundamentally to search for life, in a way that is not always conscious and is consequently dangerous. Flirting with this type of partner eventually ends in a union with death.

A society that evades the reality of death and ageing (transforming) is a sick society. A physician or caregiver who denies this reality will have difficulties caring for a dying person until the end. Any negation is a tension, a suffering that will be perceived by the patient and that works against the relationship.

13.2.3 Life as a Dynamic Force, Energy, or Vitality and Creative Principle

The vitality of life is the "vital wind", considered by 18th-century physiologists to be the cause of life itself.

13.2.3.1 Movement

Life is movement. Human cells are multiplied and this multiplication requires some vitality. Human beings are endowed with a vitality that varies throughout their life and decreases progressively with age, illness, death and suffering. For example, a mother who loses a child will often feel utter and complete exhaustion. Life is linked with wind, the respiratory function. The expression "his breathing is shallow" translates in common language as loss of vitality. The importance of wind and breath is largely underestimated in our modern world. However, throughout their lifespan, human beings are related to the surrounding world through breathing. The way a human being breathes will signify the level of harmony reached in one's life. There is a link between the respiratory quality and the response that we give to the surrounding world. Knowing how to breathe will help in relating to one's suffering and that of others.

13.2.3.2 Emergence and Resorption

This vitality exists before the conception of the human egg. The vitality that we have today already existed within the ovum and spermatozoon from which we derive. We can also observe a kind of hierarchy in the structuring, elaboration, and composition of a human being. However, this hierarchy is also observed at the other end of the chain, in a reverse way, through the process of destructuring and decomposition.

Even in the case of a brutal death, life does not leave us quickly. The process of death is slow and progressive, rather than instantaneous and brutal. The death of a human being is neither the death of the cells (after death, the hair, body hair and nails continue to grow), nor the death of the mineral substance. It is easy to confuse life and Life. The end of the existence of a human being is not the end of the life process. In terms of atomic physics, it is more realistic to envision death as a process of transformation.

In the same way that a wave is born out of the ocean and is never separated from it, human life is born out of Life and is never separated from it.

The difficulty is in the fact that we really have to experience this by ourselves. From a practical point of view, the simple and intellectual understanding of this reality is a source of great importance and ease in the relationship with the suffering and dying person.

13.2.3.3 The Vagueness of Birth and Death

As a physician caring for human beings, it is important to reflect on the origin and the end of existence, with the objective of better understanding leading to better care. We can say that a "vague zone" surrounds the birth and death of a human being. Who, it may be asked, is born and who is it that dies? This question should be at the core of the medical scientific approach and part of the research of all genuine philosophy and metaphysics.

The human egg created at the time of conception undergoes a series of successive cleavages into smaller cells, the blastomeres, which give the egg the aspect of a blackberry or morula. Up to the moment of implantation in the mucous membrane of the uterus, these cells are totipotent, capable of forming a complete embryo by themselves. This property of the preimplanted embryo progressively disappears when the embryo is implanted. The cells then develop the specificity to become tissues, organs, and so on. We do not know when we cross the line from a cluster of cells with human potentiality to a potential human being. Where is the border? It is the same for death. The famous physician, Richet, said: "Nothing is more uncertain than the moment of death". Acknowledging these realities allows us to be more flexible when viewing the situation.

To use the metaphor of the wave again, when are we able to talk about a wave and when is the wave no more? Life is movement and continuity.

Feeling this allows us to be inscribed in the natural order and dynamics of things. This vision is deeply vivifying and ensures a sense of security. It lessens the feeling of separation and softens the pain of grief. It has the power to transform radically relationships with others.

13.2.3.4 Energy

Today, the word "energy" often has rather negative impact, particularly in the context of the "New Age". The energetic dimension of a relationship is never talked about in scientific medical circles. Very simply, however, we may observe the reality of the drive for life in its many variations in our daily experience. These variations might be expressed in terms of intensity or quality, for example, the intensity of the energy of football supporters watching their own team play, or the quality of energy felt during a religious recital. This energetic dimension must be taken seriously in caring for suffering people and in listening. It is necessary to learn how to pinpoint a person's vital intensity and quality. This is a key factor of listening and one of the essential elements of the quality of Presence, which I shall discuss later.

13.3 Tridimensional Reality of Human Beings

In my experience, it is impossible to care for the sick properly without taking into account the three dimensions of the human being:

- Physical
- Psychological
- Spiritual.

There is not only an ethical or deontological problem, but also a problem of elementary logic. These three dimensions are interlocked, the negation of any one of them will only end in a partial result. They are not all affected at the same time or with the same intensity, but the three dimensions must be examined with the same rigour. For example, studies have clearly shown the relationship between an old psychological trauma and complications arising following surgery performed a long time after the traumatising event. If this psychological suffering is ignored, the outcome of the surgical procedure is at considerable risk. The sick, and particularly the cancer patient, must be heard and his or her three dimensions acknowledged. If this is done in all cases, we should be pleasantly surprised by the evolution of certain pathologies. Although we are unable to prove it, our assumption seems plausible. Even if significant improvement is not made, at least we would be in a better position to help ill people and to alleviate some of their suffering.

A human being is not only a body and a psyche (psychosomatic), he or she is also a mind:

- The somatic-corporeal (from the Greek/Latin *soma/corpus*) aspect is obvious: matter, hormones, neuromediators, etc.
- The psychological (*psukhe/anima*) aspect joins together the mental functions (thoughts, concepts, faculty of analysing, language) and the psycho-emotional functions (emotions and dreams)
- The mind-spiritual (*pneuma/spiritus*) aspect is less evident; it is also called the "cognitive" or "consciential" aspect.

It is difficult to define and understand the mind-spiritual dimension. The root of the word "spiritual" is *spiritus*, which means "mind" in the sense of "feeling": simply that which feels, knows and has experience. (This is why the term "cognitive" is used.) For example, if we bite into an apple, we will have the direct experience of tasting fruit. In the very first moment, there is a pure and naked experience of the taste of fruit. This experience, direct and simple, is derived from the mind or consciousness of the person. In the second moment, there is the elementary positioning about the taste. That which feels begins to take a position in relationship to what is felt. It is similar to an inner movement. This primitive and simple experience becomes pleasant, neutral or unpleasant. Then, the third moment consists of the conceptualisation of the experience, allowing for intervention of mental or psychological function. The experience that has been lived is named and labelled. We think, it is good or bad, sweet or sour, and so on. In reality, there is the perceiver, one who becomes conscious of the other thing and of the interaction between the perceiver and the perceived: it is pleasant or unpleasant, good or bad, and so on.

We use the term consciousness (from the Latin, *cum sciencia,* with knowledge) to define the perceiver within ourselves.

We can rightly say that this dimension of the human being is seldom, indeed never, noticed. It is completely veiled, or worse mixed up with the psychological function of the person. There is, however, a distinction. On this level, there is not only a form of suffering that needs to be acknowledged, but there is an inescapable reality of great importance in the field of relationships. Psychologists affirm that more than 60% of communication is expressed non-verbally. This corresponds more than 60% with what is felt, that is to say what the mind perceives, that which we feel.

This aspect is essential in the field of listening and in the relationship of helping. Furthermore, it is on this level that true listening is found, as we will see later.

A human being is "not a chromosomic robot, a toy in the hand of the unconscious, or a cog of social determinism," as expressed by François Brousse (poet, philosopher and metaphysician). It is a being endowed with a consciousness. We must give the consciousness, or mind, or spiritual, the place and importance that it deserves within life itself. Above all, perhaps we must consider human beings as spiritual beings endowed with the ability to think, speak and act with a body. Nevertheless, a frequent confusion often appears between the two words, spiritual and religious. It is our opinion that the function of the religious – and therefore of an authentic religion – is to link human beings, in the intimacy of their depth to this spiritual dimension and to favour the growth and nourish this profoundly human spiritual experience.

This vision is quite different from our usual modern vision of human beings. Not to account for the spiritual reality or considering it to be merely an aspect of existence among others and not the most important one, is a major aberration, from which many painful and conflicting, indeed threatening, situations in our world directly flow. This is also valid for the practice of medicine.

Negation of this dimension in any human being is not only a psychogenic factor, it may also be responsible for the fatigue syndrome or "burn out" of physicians who work in palliative care or emergency services.

13.4 What is Suffering?

Suffering can be defined as a state of discomfort or as a state of imbalance, disharmony or tension, likely to affect the physical, psychological and spiritual dimensions of human beings.

During their lives, human beings experience many sufferings linked to the nature of their constitution or to various situations. The four main causes of suffering are: birth, sickness, old age and death. There are many others, often of a psychological nature, such as not obtaining what one wishes, preserving what has been acquired, change, being separated from loved ones, or encountering unpleasant people or adverse situations. In the context of cancer or the end of human life, suffering manifests at several levels: physical, psychological, mind or consciousness, and at the vital level.

13.4.1 Suffering at the Physical Level

We use the word pain to describe suffering at the physical level. Pain is often experienced by cancer patients. It may be caused by an attack of the periosteum, irritation or ulceration of a mucous membrane, compression of a nerve, distension of a membrane or an organ, or even complications following therapy (radiotherapy, surgery, and so on).

This often chronic physical pain must be recognised as soon as it appears. It creates chronic stress for the patient, which leads to a decrease in the level of lymphocytes and a reduction in immunological function. At the therapeutic level, the more the pain is allowed to evolve, the more the patient remembers it, and it therefore becomes more difficult to treat. The persistence of pain leads to a form of exhaustion and a "living hell", destroying any communication, and confining the patient to psychological depression and prostration (psychomotor atony of the child, fetal position of the elderly, for example).

To this physical pain is generally added physical discomfort. It is not only painful, but the occasional discomfort (or disability) creates psychological suffering. Permanent itching irritates, respiratory difficulties create anxiety, nauseous sensations exhaust, and so on. The interaction of the somatic with the psychological sphere is obvious in some cases. For example, a bone metastasis will attack the periosteum, the source of bone pain, then bone destruction will produce a higher blood level of calcium (hypercalcaemia). This in turn, if not treated, will bring about a state of confusion, causing behavioural problems.

13.4.2 Suffering at the Psychological Level

At the psychological level, suffering often begins with the appearance of the first worrying symptom. The person will see a physician. Then, depending on the quality and the authenticity of the relationship, this suffering will be more or less amplified. It is difficult enough to suffer in our bodies. However, being unable to talk about it, being isolated in what we feel, and being unable to express it, aggravate this psychological suffering. Moreover, this has some consequences on the physical pain. Progressively, the illness evolves with a succession of griefs:

- Loss of health and vitality
- Loss of autonomy
- Loss of social status and role
- Loss of the body image, family role and material goods.

Loss of social status and role is often difficult to bear because of conditioning and strong social pressures that associate the notion of dignity with the notion of usefulness. "I have dignity if I am useful." The question of dignity is very important. Dignity is linked to the fact that we are living beings, that we have a spiritual dimension, that we have an ability to feel inside this space of love and light that makes us feel alive, even if we are on the verge of dying. The philosopher Christian Zundel said: "The true problem is not to know if we will live after death but if we will be alive before death." It is surprising to observe that certain disabled or dying people are sometimes much more alive than many people in "good health."

Successive losses of body image, family role, material goods, existential suffering (What is the meaning of my life now that I am bedridden?), fear of the unknown, fear of the moment of death (Is it painful at the time of dying?) and exhaustion from mental projection are associated with emotional and psychological manifestations characteristic of the process of grieving, such as denegation, denial, refusal, anger, bargaining, depression, and so on. These emotions are also seen among people close to the dying person and those who care for him or her.

13.4.3 Suffering at the Level of Mind or Consciousness

Suffering at the level of mind or consciousness is more subtle and often not clearly visible. It does exist, however, even in the absence of a specific context for severe illness or end of life. As in geology, there are many strata of suffering. For example, one may experience suffering when everything is fine, simply feeling frustration or that something is lacking. One feels separated. In a religious Christian context, it could be said that one is "out of the Father's house," divided inside. In a Buddhist context, one talks of dualism. Something is lacking for one to be fully happy and unified. This feeling to exist separately, in an individual way, is suffering itself. It is the essential spiritual suffering – or simply the suffering of the mind – activated by processes of separation, whatever they are. Death materialises the ultimate separation, bares to the bones, strips this suffering or fundamental tension that is veiled most of the time. It is at the root of psychological behaviour observed during separation. And when we talk about stress, it is also there that we find its source.

Finally, all the griefs of our lives and much of our suffering point only in this direction. Suffering does not have to be sought out, it occurs anyway, quickly and without being invoked. Its utility may possibly lead the receptive human being in the right direction, that of Life beyond all sufferings.

13.4.4 Suffering at the Vital Level

Illness, old age and the end of life are often characterised by a decrease in vitality. Lacking the strength to walk, to raise the hand from the surface of the bed, or even to inhale normally are sources of suffering for the person experiencing them. Suddenly, one feels vulnerable and fragile. This awareness of our fragility could create pain and even anxiety.

13.5 Caring for Suffering People

Even professionals find it difficult to confront suffering, particularly the suffering associated with the problems of a serious illness, end of life and death. The suffering of others may mirror our own sufferings and difficulties.

The words "cancer" and "metastasis" are frequently vectors of images of death. Caring for these patients is difficult because of the increased awareness of the reality of death.

Caring is part of the framework of the relationship of helping and tending. It must pacify and suppress, or at least decrease, the painful tension at each level. The word "therapist" means "the one who accompanies on a path". The caregiver or the volunteer is the one who accompanies others on their difficult path to prevent them from falling. The Greek word *therapeuo* means serving, caring for and worshipping, i.e. cultivating and also caring. The role of the caregiver (including the physician) is not to cure, but to suppress and soothe suffering, through healing if possible. A patient does not come to see a physician saying "Doctor, operate on my appendicitis," he or she comes because of stomach aches. If we confuse caring and curing, we end up excluding those who cannot be cured, such as disabled people and the elderly, which is unacceptable from an ethical and humane point of view.

13.5.1 Various Modalities of Caring

13.5.1.1 Caring for the Body

Caring for the body is characterised by efficient treatment of pain and symptoms inherent to the end of life, in a way that provides comfort for the patient. This is associated with careful nursing, using massage and a bath whenever possible. Caring for the body is indispensable in approaching deeper layers of suffering. The therapeutic approach is logical. First, we treat the most obvious painful layers and move toward the more subtle and profound ones. This entails solid professional competence and knowledge on the part of the caregivers.

13.5.1.2 Caring for the Psyche

Caring for the psyche means helping others to mature psychologically, to accept the reality and to transform this ordeal, which was not chosen, into a maturing experience. To quote Zundel: "In fact, it is a matter for the one that assists powerless to the biological destruction of the other, to recognise in the other, this inner human being, in order to make him or her aware of it." This awareness is accompanied by work on the emotions. Serious illness and the end of life are moments of crisis, generating expressed or repressed emotions. Therefore, it is important to help the emotional expression of the ill person, because too much emotional tension prevents analysis and accordingly decreases the patient's understanding of the situation. Hence, it is necessary that the caregiver understands as much as possible what others are experiencing. One patient was heard to say about the caregivers around him: "If only they could try to understand me." This work requires from the caregiver, permanent staff or volunteer, some knowledge and an understanding of the functional mechanisms of the human psyche, his or hers in particular, in order to see the reality more precisely.

The way we see the world and others is often filtered through a mental prism. This prism is made heavier by the contents of the memory, such as preconceived ideas, fears, a priori, and so on, which veil the reality. We experience what we are and we are what we experience. Our experiences form us. When our vision sheds its past – mental images, projections and remnants – a new understanding appears, based not on acquired knowledge but on direct perception of what really is. It is what Jung said when he spoke of "withdrawing projections". We cannot help others beyond the level to which we have helped ourselves. Indeed, how can we understand, within the other, what is eluded within us? In the same way, knowledge and that which has been lived by communication and relaxation (being relaxed means being free of tensions) are not useless (transactional analysis, neurolinguistic programming, analytic method, sophrology, and so on).

Finally, being truthful with the patient is essential and merits a particular development. Two questions may be posed:

- What is truth?
- How do we share what we know with the patient?

The answer to the first question could be that truth is simply what is, the face of reality, and that it is valid only in the present moment. The notion of living day to day with ill people is important and requires some flexibility, as far as the prognostics are concerned.

In effect, prognostics are elaborated from statistics, which are established from groups of individuals. However, what is valid for a group is not necessarily valid for any given individual. Too much emphasis on the prognosis risks veiling the real situation of the ill person; it may even cause aggression. We may "condemn" or sometimes "save" ill people before investigating the real situation. This can even sometimes hinder a favorable evolution of the illness. The projection, whether negative or positive, is always aggressive for the person who receives it, all the more so since the perception of what is not said is very acute for the seriously ill or dying person. Intuition is enhanced when other functions have disappeared.

As for the second question, sharing the truth requires the physician to overcome personal obstacles, such as his or her own fear and anxiety about facing illness or death. He or she must develop humane qualities and particularly the ability to listen. Three points are important in approaching truth:

- Trust
- The right attitude
- Sensitivity and intuition to allow decoding and deciphering.

When we have lied once, it is difficult to recover the trust of an ill person. Trust is an essential element of therapy. We should be sufficiently subtle never to lie to the ill person. At the same time, we must adapt to his or her desire to know, and be aware that this person is not always ready to hear the truth. The patient should be allowed to approach his or her truth, not ours, through an open attitude, that is to say to let him or her evolve progressively toward the information by honestly answering the questions asked, at the moment chosen by the ill person to ask them.

Giving information that has not been requested too early or refusing it at the time it is requested is a source of anxiety. Sensitivity and intuition are required to allow decoding and deciphering; this is the art of seeing what is behind the words and pain, i.e. listening.

Finally, caring for the ill person also implicates caring for the close friends and family. Caring for the family has an indirect therapeutic effect on the patient, because of the attachment between them. It is an important part of the work of a caregiver.

13.5.1.3 Caring for the Mind

Here, we are particularly concerned with the subtle act of listening. Under normal circumstances, we understand listening to be essentially at the psychological level. However, the listening that we are talking about here – even if it includes the psychological aspect – has greater profundity. It has two dimensions: comprehending and therapeutic.

Comprehending listening is the art of becoming aware of what is behind the words. It is the most profound and genuine level of comprehension, a true incorporation (the verb comprehend comes from the Latin *cum prehendere,* which means *taking into oneself, inside oneself*).

Therapeutic listening is listening that heals. It induces within the patient a relaxation and hence a relief of the suffering. Such listening requires the caregiver to develop certain qualities.

13.5.2 Qualities and Competence of the Caregiver

When we face the suffering of others, it is difficult to find the correct attitude (the right words and behaviour) without letting ourselves be destroyed by what is said or seen. This is a major preoccupation of caregivers, as I have pointed out earlier.

"Modern man has a hard heart and tender guts," said the theologist Bernanos. Hard heart, because he or she remains indifferent to others' suffering (denial); soft guts, because if this suffering is perceived, he or she is unable to handle it. Therefore, it is necessary to develop a good heart and strong guts, creating an inner strength, union of kindness and gentleness, acute perception or rightness of feeling and inner stability.

Emergence of these essential qualities is associated with developing the four interdependent aspects (physical, psychological, spiritual and vital) in the caregiver.

13.5.2.1 Physical Aspects

Caregivers need to overcome any narcissistic attitudes they might have to their bodies. They should understand that the body can teach them something. We must begin by examining everything we do in our relationship with our body, psyche and mind, and truly "become friends" with our body. We must develop the ability to feel, getting the sensation in our body and understand where the body is an instrument of union and communication and where it becomes an instrument of cutting and separating.

The role of breathing, the exact perception of the true gravity centre, and the position of the body are fundamental. For example, the position of kneeling with joined palms favours a particular state of mind. The cross-legged posture with a straight back and relaxed abdomen, held for some time and corrected regularly, has the power to calm mental function and reinforce psychological stability. When we want to listen deeply, it is important to be stable and relaxed internally.

The correct diet (good quality and the correct quantity) is important (caregivers often eat poorly). The frequency of ingestion must be respected (eating should be related to appetite and not frustration). Bodily health is important. The flexibility of the body should not be neglected, and sufficient sleep is necessary.

13.5.2.2 Psychological Aspects

Psychological aspects in a relationship are numerous. It is necessary to develop a calm and serene mind by progressively developing an ability to sustain attention. This state allows emergence of three fundamental qualities: stability, clarity and openness. A mind cluttered by multiple thoughts and unceasing mental wanderings are serious obstacles to listening.

Freedom relating to our emotions and projections is also essential. There are two classical ways to deal with the emotions: expression and suppression. There is another less used way, which consists of simply witnessing the emotion (emotion is neither followed nor suppressed, it is simply acknowledged and not grasped). This ability depends on a particular way of training the mind, which leads to a deeper understanding of its functioning. This requires developing some clarity: becoming aware that we are implicated in an emotional and/or projecting process, and then developing the ability to not identify with it by not grasping it. This stability, clear and open, is a source of great benefit, notably creating inner peace and physical ease. It is a form of contemplative experience.

Finally, this work on oneself requires the alert sensitivity of a child and the humbleness of a searching student who tries to learn and discover without imposing subjective attitude and reactions. One must furthermore show some courage and a sense of responsibility to live honestly with what is learned, independently from the consequences.

13.5.2.3 Aspects of Awareness

Usually, we identify strongly with our thoughts and emotions. As stated earlier, it is possible through training the mind to be less dependent on our own thoughts and emotions and to become more free from the "spontaneous" mechanism called "egoistical grasping," and less dependent on the operation of grasping. This greater freedom creates a space, an opening endowed with more availability and receptivity; to be available for others and receptive to others' suffering. Genuine Presence resides in a true absence and giving up the will of the "I"or ego.

This experience of Presence is that of more flexible and relaxed attention, which is a kind of permanent listening. The presence of an intelligence that is not affected by the mental ego allows emergence of the best possible response to the situation. This is a state of no fear, a calm that releases a great strength for handling a situation (strength in the meaning of an inner force, not strength favouring manipulation of others or the situation).

In this context, situations are not apprehended through fear and pleasure, but integrated in a totality. It is here that there is true listening, the deepest listening. Listening is totally independent from mental function while giving a greater harmony to it.

13.5.2.4 Vital Aspects

Generally, we waste our vitality in non-essential secondary things. This waste tires and troubles us at the end of the day. We must discover our true priorities in life, discovering the order of these priorities and harmoniously dividing up our time and energy in this order. (Beware of the time thieves!) Each movement of the body, each thought, each emotion and each concept uses vitality. Our education begins with observing how to use this vitality by learning how not to lose it through various attitudes such as gossiping, excitability, fear, and so on. In the same way, at a deeper level, the experience of lesser grasping is a source of greater vitality and also the source of greater sensitivity. Not grasping thoughts and emotions saves energy that can be used in other ways, leading to more subtle functioning of the body and mind. Furthermore, at the level of relationships, it is important to appreciate together the intensity of the vitality of a person as well as the quality of his or her vitality. The quality of this vitality helps in some ways to find the level of the relationship, seeing the energy activated in the situation and/or in the relationship and being capable to "dance with it." Finally, it is being in harmony and resonating with the situation.

13.6 Conclusion

Relieving a living being from suffering is of great importance. It is included in the caregiver's ethics and requires commitment and strong motivation. We often have the tendency to forget that our main function is to suppress, indeed to relieve, suffering, whether by curing it whenever possible through a curative approach, or caring though a palliative approach. Listening to suffering requires specific humane qualities that we must develop, such as opening, clarity and Presence. Presence includes genuine love and compassion. They are sources of harmony for the caregivers and for the sick. It is not a matter of being perfect, but of being able to understand our perfectibility.

As caregivers, we know that our skill to extend our help depends on our inner state. Human beings are thrown off balance by experiencing great suffering. They become very vulnerable. Finding themselves surrounded by competent people, an atmosphere of gentleness, kindness and non-aggressiveness will be something to lean on in their disarray. As caregivers, it is our obligation to give the patient such an environment.

For the sick, the relationship established with illness, or even the way he or she lives the illness is of great importance. It is strongly desirable for the ill person to establish a sane relationship with illness and to accept what it is. In this atmosphere of accepting, illness has less ascendancy: "it has nothing to feed on." The possibilities of improvement become greater. Physicians should teach patients the correct attitude to allow them to establish the most harmonious relationship with their situation. It is not easy, but it is a important part of the art of caring.

Finally, an understanding of what is death, and also life, is intimately linked to an understanding of what is consciousness, of what we are in essence, and of the knowledge we have of ourselves. "The relationship we establish with death depends on the depth in which we are rooted." A better understanding of life, birth, death and suffering comes with spiritual ripening, with the blossoming of the spiritual dimension of a Human Being. We accept the expansion of the body and the ripening of the psyche, why not that of the consciousness?

For some years, we have considered the physical suffering of ill people. We have only recently become aware that the sick can think, have emotions and feelings; and that we should accompany them on the psycho-affective path. However, this is far from being practised everywhere. The next step is to consider the mind of the sick. This step that must begin today in order to continue tomorrow. It is unfortunate, but understandable, that this dimension of Reality is so infrequently approached in medical seminars (it is merely touched upon during seminars on palliative care and most often in a superficial manner). This work is delicate because it requires developing a knowledge that has no reference in other knowledge, a knowledge that transcends all knowledge. This requires dismissal of a dogmatic and marked attitude, which most of us find difficult.

Part 7

Pain Relief

14 Therapeutic Approaches to Bone Cancer Pain

M. Baciuchka-Palmaro, J.L. Mouysset and D. Spiegel

14.1 Introduction

Pain is one of the major symptoms of bone cancer. In 1984, 19 million cancer patients around the world suffered pain (Elliot and Foley, 1989). The prevalence of cancer pain is an important problem, as 30% of patients receiving curative treatment and 70% of patients with palliative care suffer pain because of the progression of the tumour (Greenwald et al, 1987).

The pathophysiology of cancer pain is variable, according to the invasion or compression of several tissues (visceral, somatic and nervous structures).

The prevalence and intensity of cancer pain depend on the tumour type, the stage of disease progression, the presence of metastases, the treatment and the presence of concurrent anxiety or depression. Bone and pancreatic cancers are the most painful, whatever the degree of disease progression (Table 14.1).

14.2 Bone Metastases and Pain

In 30–70% of cancer patients, bone metastases are diagnosed. They may induce several kinds of pain: vertebral pain, base of skull syndromes, or diffuse or focal bone pain of the long bones, chest wall, etc.).

Table 14.1. Prevalence of cancer pain. From Bonica and Loeser (1990)

Tumour	Stage of disease	Prevalence (%)
Bone	Advanced	75–80 (70–85)
Pancreas	Advanced	79 (72–100)
Stomach	Advanced	75 (67–77)
Colon	Advanced	69 (47–95)
Breast	Advanced	72 (56–94)
Prostate	Advanced	75 (40–100)
Uterus	Advanced	70 (55–80)
Lung	Advanced	72 (58–85)
Lymphoma	Advanced	58 (20–69)
Leukaemia	Advanced	52 (5–58)
All	Advanced	50 (11–75)
All	All stages	71 (52–96)

Bone metastases can also involve compression or infiltration of the peripheral or central nervous system, or sensory or motor deficiencies.

14.2.1 Vertebral Pain Syndromes

Bone metastases are often located in the vertebrae. Characteristics of the pain depend on the metastatic sites (Table 14.2).

14.2.2 Base of Skull Metastases

Base of skull metastases can appear as a result of progression of breast, prostatic or head and neck cancer. Some localisations lead to headache or cranial nerve symptoms (frontal, orbital, ethmoidal, sphenoidal). There may be associated neurological problems, such as diplopia, sensory deficiency or trigeminal paralysis.

14.2.3 Diffuse Bone Pain

Diffuse bone pain is often the most important and requires systemic treatment. It commonly arises from breast, lung, prostate, thyroid and kidney cancers.

14.2.4 Long Bone Metastases

These metastases induce acute pain when the extremity is subjected to tension, and pain should lead to the suspicion of bone fracture.

Table 14.2. Vertebral pain. From De Conno and Caraceni (1996)

Vertebrae	Pain characteristics	Notes
C1–C2	Neck pain radiating to the vertex, acute with exion/extension of neck	Cord compression at cervico-medullary junction. Dissociated nervous syndrome
C3–C4	Neck pain radiating to shoulders	
C5–C6	Neck, shoulder, arm pain	Often associated with radiculopathy
C7–D1	Interscapular pain, arm pain	Same as C5–C6
Dorsal	Middle dorsal pain can radiate to the chest	When bilateral, tight band-like sensation, compression fracture very likely with epidural extension
T12–L1	Groin pain radiating to the genitals	In case of radiculopathy can be elicited by neck exion
L2	Low back pain, upper thigh	
L3	Low back pain, upper and external area of the thigh, knee	
L4–L5	Low back pain, pain below knee	Sudden increase of pain with impossibility of moving indicates vertebral body compression fracture
S1–S2	Sacral pain, posterior thigh, popliteal fossa	
S3–S5	Sacral pain, gluteal and perineal	Cauda equina compression main complication

14.2.5 Epidural Spinal Cord Compression

Epidural spinal cord compression is the most dangerous complication of vertebral metastases. It occurs in 5–10% of patients with cancer. When it appears, the quality of life of patients is reduced substantially. Epidural spinal cord compression leads to paraplegia or quadriplegia without treatment. The relative risk of epidural extension and therefore of cord compression must be evaluated before any treatment (De Conno and Caraceni, 1996).

14.3 Management of Bone Pain

The medical priority is sustained pain relief by permanent treatment, whatever the degree of disease progression. Specific and continuous treatment must always be initiated as soon as curative care begins.

14.3.1 Surgical treatment

Tumour resection and bone consolidation are the two major surgical methods used to treat bone metastases. Additional radiotherapy is usually recommended in palliative care.

The different indications are risk of fracture, flat bone or long bone fracture, vertebral instability or epidural spinal cord compression.

14.3.1.1 Risk of Fracture

Risk of fracture is higher when the diameter of osteolytic lesions is greater than or equal to 2.5 cm on the lower limb bones. Fracture occurs in 50% of cases if at least half of the cortical area is affected (Fidler, 1981). The high occurrence of fractures in long bones is a reason to establish preventive treatment.

14.3.1.2 Fractures

Surgery is the only way to set a pathological fracture. Additional radiotherapy leads to secondary consolidation in 70% of cases (Durandeau and Genste, 1989).

14.3.1.3 Vertebral metastases

Spinal vertebrae are the most frequent sites of bone metastases (Clain, 1965). Variable pain intensity is due to the level of bone invasion (periosteal invasion, spinal instability, spinal compression or fracture, epidural or nervous invasion). Radiotherapy and additional external setting are indicated. In the case of one vertebral lytic lesion, without posterior extension, percutaneous injection of alcohol is recommended.

Surgery remains the major treatment in the event of neurological symptoms, persistent pain or increasing vertebral deformation. In these cases, additional radiotherapy is indicated. Radiotherapy with corticotherapy is preferred when more than three vertebrae are affected or if the tumour has good radiosensitivity.

14.3.2 Radiation Therapy

Whatever the primary tumour, bone metastases are particularly sensitive to radiotherapy. Most analgesic effects are obtained after 4 weeks, after which analgesic drugs may be added.

However, metabolic radiotherapy seems to be less useful in diffuse and multiple bone localisations. Analgesia is usually obtained in 14 days. This kind of radiation therapy is being evaluated in myelomas, lymphomas, breast and prostate cancers (Turner et al, 1989).

14.3.3 Specific Treatment

The specific treatments (chemotherapy, endocrine therapy, immunotherapy, gene therapy) must be considered as primary interventions for pain in acute care. In palliative care, patients can live without symptoms and the side-effects do not affect the quality of life all the time. These specific treatments may decrease the threshold of pain in 75% of suffering patients. Common indications for specific treatments to relieve pain are bone metastases of lung cancer, multiple myeloma, breast cancer, prostate cancer, sarcomas and melanomas (Krakowski, 1996).

Management of cancer pain is not separate from treatment. The difficulty is to distinguish palliative from terminal cancer care (Krakowski et al, 1995).

14.3.4 Pharmacological Pain Management

The use of analgesic drugs can bring relief to 90% of cancer patients. However, 10% of patients need invasive techniques (anaesthetic and neurosurgical techniques) to achieve adequate analgesia (World Health Organization, 1996).

The "three-step analgesic ladder" of the World Health Organization (WHO) is recommended for the management of cancer pain. The indications are to deliver different analgesic treatment in accordance with intensity of pain in a stepwise fashion (Table 14.3). The optimal response will be obtained after 24–48 hours' treatment, depending on drug dosages.

14.3.4.1 Analgesic Drugs

The WHO describes five main principles of analgesic prescription:

- Oral route of administration
- Fixed hour prescriptions
- The three-step analgesic ladder

Table 14.3. The three-step analgesic ladder of the World Health Organization

PAIN	
↓	
STEP 1:	Non-opioid
	± Adjuvant
↓	
PAIN PERSISTING OR INCREASING	
↓	
STEP 2:	Opioid for mild to moderate pain
	± Non-opioid
	± Adjuvant
↓	
PAIN PERSISTING OR INCREASING	
↓	
STEP 3:	Opioid for moderate to severe pain
	± Non-opioid
	± Adjuvant
↓	
FREEDOM FROM CANCER PAIN	

- Individual prescriptions
- Detailed prescriptions.

14.3.4.2 Three-step Analgesic Ladder

Non-opioid drugs are recommended in the first step of the WHO analgesic ladder, to relieve mild to moderate pain. Non-steroidal anti-inflammatory drugs (NSAIDs) or paracetamol are usually used. The recommendation of noramidopyrine for pain management is a matter of debate because of major medullary toxicity.

At step 2 of the WHO analgesic ladder, when cancer pain cannot be relieved using NSAIDs, patients should receive additional opioid regimens for moderate to severe pain, such as codeine and oxycodeine. They can be used in single preparations or combined with other analgesics, such as acetaminophen, aspirin or paracetamol. Propoxyphene and meperidine are usually administered, but the prescription of meperidine is controversial because of central nervous system toxicity with parenteral doses.

At step 3 of the WHO analgesic ladder, for severe pain or inadequate analgesia with a sound step 2 drug, oral morphine regimens are required. The dosing guidelines are described in Table 14.4.

Alternative routes of administration, when the oral route is unsuitable or inadvisable because of side-effects, are as follows:

- Continuous infusions (subcutaneous or intravenous) are used in patients who have dysphagia, nausea and vomiting with oral opioids, gastrointestinal obstruction, excessive side-effects with parenteral bolus administration, or inadequate analgesia relief with oral morphine
- Spinal opioid administration is required when side-effects of systemic therapy occur
- Transdermal administration with "patches" of fentanyl is comfortable and convenient for the cancer patient (Miser et al, 1989). The efficacy seems to be equal

Table 14.4. Oral morphine dosing guidelines. From De Conno and Caraceni (1996)

Establish initial dose	Opioid-naive patient: start with 5–10 mg morphine every 4 h or equivalent Slow-release morphine should be started at 10 mg every 12 h in most patients; higher initial dosing can be tried only with expert advice
Titrate dose to effect	Increase total daily dose to at least 30–50% of previous dose every 24 h until pain relief satisfactory or excessive unmanageable side-effects occur Maximum recommended dose is immaterial, individual variability can be > ten-fold
Fixed dosing around the clock in accordance with the serum half-life of each analgesic	In most patients with cancer it is necessary and allows pain relief and night-time sleep, preventing pain reoccurrence
As-needed dosing	Pain relief is often uneven and breakthrough pain is very common; always provide doses with a short-acting opioid every 2 h. Doses should be equal to 5–15% of daily requirements
Management of side-effects	Explain to the patient that side-effects are potential but not unavoidable, and manageable Always give prophylactic therapy for constipation only

to that of oral morphine and the incidence of gastrointestinal toxicity is less (Korte et al, 1996)

- The rectal route of administration is indicated to relieve pain after or in combination with other oral or parenteral routes
- Sublingual and buccal administration is preferred for treating moderate pain with buprenorphine (De Conno et al, 1993) and fentanyl (Fine et al, 1991). When no or insufficient analgesic response is obtained with opioids, adjuvant analgesics should be used to relieve opioid-resistant pain.

Adjuvant analgesics, such as corticosteroids, antidepressants (tricyclic or selective serotonin reuptake inhibitors), anticonvulsive drugs, oral local anaesthetics and anticholinergic drugs, are usually used in combination with opioid or analgesic drugs at step 3 of the analgesic ladder.

Biphosphonates play a major role, particularly in bone disease and pain (Tubiana-Hulin, 1996). Clodronate and pamidronate are often prescribed for pain. Pain relief may be obtained in 30–50% of patients receiving intravenous clodronate. The analgesic efficacy of pamidronate is dose-dependent (Berenson et al, 1996). Efficient doses seem to be 3-weekly regimens of 90 mg intravenously. Oral clodronate is a good maintenance treatment.

14.3.5 Non-pharmacological Pain Management

In most cases, drugs used for inflammatory disease are efficient and eliminate or reduce the pain to a level where it is not a major concern to the patient. With bone metastasis, pain may be acute (fracture) or chronic, and despite advances in the pharmacological management of both types of pain, strictly pharmacological management is often not sufficient. Pain changes throughout the day, and with activity. Even anti-inflammatory drug and opiate, and/or chemotherapy/metabolic or classical radiotherapy may not completely control pain. Moreover, these treatments have significant side-effects. Some patients therefore require a more global approach to pain management, beyond pharmacological treatment.

Pain is the ultimate psychosomatic phenomenon. Thus, while physical disruption by tumour invasion may be associated with pain, only about one-third of such patients experience moderate pain. Pain is a frequent but not universal symptom: lesions at the same sites sometimes result in pain and sometimes do not. Clearly, the psychological reactive component has a major determining effect in the pain experience of some patients. Central to this is the theoretical division of the pain experience into two components: the sensation of the painful stimulus itself and the reactive component to it. This was established clinically by Beecher (1956), when he observed that the experience of pain and demands for pain medication were proportional to the meaning of the pain experience rather to the extent of the tissue damage. For example, soldiers wounded on the Anzio beachhead in World War II demanded far less pain medication than a less seriously injured group of surgical patients at Massachusetts General Hospital.

Several somatic and psychological variables influence the degree and threshold of pain sensation: muscle tension, depression, anxiety related to the pain, the amount of attention given to it by both patient and family, and the secondary gain it may offer.

14.3.5.1 Muscle tension

Muscle tension is often a component of pain sensation, and can easily be diminished by relaxation, which is the first step of hypnosis. Hypnosis can be defined as aroused attentive focal concentration with a concomitant constriction of peripheral awareness. Hypnosis (and self-hypnosis) may also help the patient to alter the meaning of the pain, and has itself an analgesic action by enhancing inhibitory processes in the nervous system.

14.3.5.2 Depression and anxiety

Depression and anxiety frequently co-occur with pain: chronic pain is itself depressing, because of the discomfort and its symbolic function as a reminder of the disease presence and process, and its associated threat to the quality and quantity of life. Furthermore, depressed patients are less able to cope with pain, so the pain sensation is increased with depression. Thus, diagnosis and treatment of depression with antidepressant medication and brief psychotherapy can be extremely effective in both treating the depression and reducing the pain; that usually requires higher doses of antidepressants, used by themselves in lower doses as pain treatment.

14.3.5.3 Meaning of the pain

As indicated above, it has been established that the meaning of pain affects its intensity. Beecher (1956) showed that the meaning of the pain was a stronger factor in determining pain intensity than was the extent of tissue damage. Seen from this perspective, whatever the balance of physical and psychological factors, the first step is acknowledging the patient's discomfort, no matter what its source. The most frequent fears associated with pain are fears of disability, death, loss of physical control and social isolation. These fears may lose power with the provision of information, better patient–physician communication, individual psychotherapy and supportive–expressive group therapy (Woodforde and Fielding, 1970; Trijsburg et al, 1992; Spiegel and Bloom, 1983b).

14.3.5.4 Secondary gain

Patients may amplify the pain signals for unconscious or conscious reasons, such as economic gain (litigation with insurance) or social reinforcement (many patients use their complaints as a way of obtaining attention and concern, as well as medication) (Holland, 1993; Table 14.5).

14.4 Conclusion

Surgery, radiotherapy, specific treatments and psycho-oncological approaches can all relieve metastatic bone pain. The indications depend on the primary tumour,

Table 14.5. Adjunctive psychosocial treatment strategies for pain control

Pain perception restructuring
Training in self-hypnosis
Behavioural family interventions
Placebo
Treatment of affective disorders
Depression: psychotherapy (group and individual)
antidepressants
Anxiety: psychotherapy (group and individual)
benzodiazepines
biofeedback
self-hypnosis
Treatment of cognitive problems
Pain-related fears
psychotherapy (group and individual)
improved communication with primary physician
rehabilitation approach to overcoming disability
Psychotic delusions
antipsychotics
Social problems
Isolation
problem-focussed group support
family consultation or therapy
Secondary gain
family consultation or therapy
rapid resolution of pending legal proceedings
Reinforcement of pain-related behaviour
family consultation or therapy
behavioural paradigm (positive reinforcement for non-pain-related behaviour)

degree of bone invasion, functional risks and the performance status of patient quality of life, concurrent anxiety and depression and prognosis.

References

Beecher HK (1956) Relationship of significance of wound to pain experienced. *JAMA* 161:1609–1613.

Berenson JR, Lichenstein A, Porter L et al (1996) Efficacy of pamidronate in reducing skeletal events in patients with advanced multiple myeloma. N Engl J Med 334:488–493.

Bonica JJ, Loeser JD (1990) Medical evaluation of the patient with pain. In: Bonica JJ, Loeser JD, Chapman CR et al (eds) The management of pain, 2nd edn. Lea & Febiger, Pennsylvania, pp 563–580.

Clain A (1965) Secondary malignant disease of bone. Br J Cancer 19:5.

De Conno F, Caraceni A (1996) Manual of cancer pain. pp 19.

De Conno F, Ripamonti C, Sbanotto A et al (1993) A clinical note on sublingual buprenorphine. J Palliative Care 9:44–46.

Durandeau A, Genste R (1989) Traitement chirurgical des fractures métastatiques et des métastases des os longs. A propos de 73 cas. Revue de Chirurgie Orthopédique et Réparatrice de l'Appareil Locomoteur 75:1–10.

Elliot K, Foley KM (1989) Neurologic pain syndromes in patients with cancer. Neurol Clin 7:333–360.

Erickson MH (1959) Hypnosis in painful terminal illness. Am J Clin Hypn 1:117–121.

Fidler M (1981) Incidence of fractures through metastases in long bones. Acta Orthop Scand 52:623–627.

Fine PG, Marcus M, DeBoer AJ et al (1991) An open label study of oral transmucosal fentanyl citrate (OTFC) for the treatment of breakthrough cancer pain. Pain 45:149–155.

Greenwald HP, Bonica JJ, Bergner M (1987) The prevalence of pain in four cancers. Cancer 60:2563–2569.

Holland JC (1993) Principles of psychooncology. In: Holland JC, Frei E (eds) Cancer medicine, 3rd edn. Lea & Febiger, Philadelphia, pp 1017–1033.

Holroyd J (1996) Hypnosis treatment of clinical pain: understanding why hypnosis is useful. Int J Clin Exp Hypn XLIV(1):33–51.

Korte W, De Stoutz N, Morant R (1996) Day-to-day titration to initiate transdermal fentanyl in patients with cancer pain: short- and long-term experiences in a prospective study of 39 patients. J Pain Symptom Management 11:139–146.

Krakowski I (1996) Chirurgie, radiotherapie et traitements médicaux spécifiques dans la prise en charge de la douleur cancéreuse. In: European School of Oncology (eds) Douleur et cancer, pp 51–68.

Krakowski I, Falcoff H, Gestin Y et al (1995) Recommandations pour une bonne pratique dans la prise en charge de la douleur du cancer chez l'adulte et l'enfant. Opération «Standards, Options et Recommandations» en cancérologie de la Fédération Nationale des Centres de Lutte Contre Le Cancer. Bulletin du Cancer 82(suppl 4):244–315.

Miser AW, Narang PK, Dothge JA et al (1989) Transdermal fentanyl for pain control in patients with cancer. Pain 37:15–21.

Sacerdote P (1980) Hypnosis and terminal illness. In: Burroughs GD, Dennerstein L (eds) Handbook of hypnosis and psychosomatic medicine. Elsevier/North-Holland Biomedical Press, New York.

Spiegel D (1981) Hypnosis in the treatment of psychosomatic symptoms and pain. Psychiatric Ann 11(9):24–30.

Spiegel D, Bloom JR (1983a) Pain in metastatic breast cancer. Cancer 52:341–345.

Spiegel D, Bloom JR (1983b) Group therapy and hypnosis reduce metastatic breast carcinoma pain. Psychosom Med 45:333–339.

Trijsburg RW, Van Knippenberg FCE, Rijpma SE (1992) Effects of psychological treatment on cancer patients: a critical review. Psychosom Med 54:489–517.

Tubiana-Hulin M (1996) Traitements médicaux des métastases osseuses. Bulletin du Cancer/Radiothérapie 83:299–304.

Turner JH, Claringbold PG, Hetherington EL (1989) A phase I study of samarium-153 ethylnediaminetetramethylene phosphonate therapy for disseminated skeletal metastases. J Clin Oncol 7:1926–1931.

Woodforde JM, Fielding JR (1970) Pain and cancer. J Psychosom Res 14:365–370.

World Health Organization (1996) Cancer pain relief, 2nd edn. World Health Organization, Geneva.

Conclusion

by D.G. Poitout

Advances in surgical techniques over the past decade have changed dramatically the prognosis of patients with bone metastases, leading to a significant improvement in overall survival and quality of life. On the other hand, although progress in the field of adult oncology has been constant, it has not been dramatic.

However, it is known that patients treated for sarcomas during the 1980s will be obtaining higher curative rates and better living conditions than those treated in any other decade in the past. Each institution has developed its own approach to the treatment of metastatic bone tumours. These treatment protocols are based on the experience and skills of the individuals, in association with the technological resources available. The application of the different steps in each treatment programme has been designed to obtain the best result for each treatment modality. The results obtained are based on a disciplined multidisciplinary effort, which can be considered as an institutional achievement.

Progress in cytogenetic knowledge has allowed a new approach for tumour classification.

When surgery was considered the only method of treatment, the survival rate was no greater than 20%. With the introduction of chemotherapy, management of tumour disease experienced an entirely new outcome. Multidisciplinary treatments that combine surgery, radiotherapy and chemotherapy show better results and a survival rate greater than 65% 5 years after diagnosis.

Today, we are challenged with a new therapeutic goal: to decrease the aggressiveness of the treatment, but at the same time, to cure the disease.

This book has discussed the experience of the contributors with treatments involving conservative surgery of the extremities, conservation of body image (salvage surgery for the limbs) and the use of new therapeutic procedures such as intra-arterial infusion of drugs and intra-operative radiotherapy for the management of malignant sarcomas.

Index